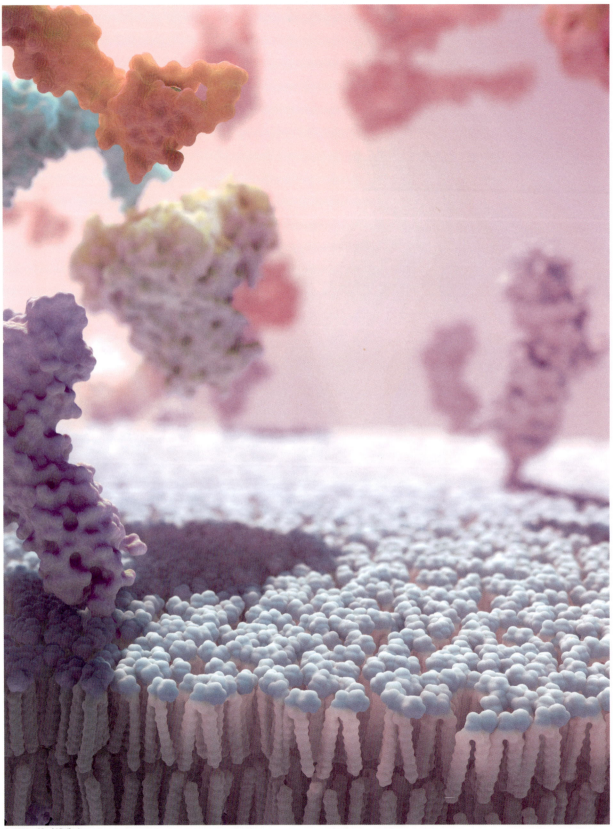

Courtesy of David Bolinsky

Neo.Life

25 Visions for the Future of Our Species

Jane Metcalfe | Brian Bergstein

Regular edition ISBN: 978-1-7331520-0-6

Library of Congress Control Number:
2019948533

Published by NEO.LIFE, Inc.
1700 Shattuck Ave. #5
Berkeley, CA 94709
Subscribe to the newsletter: www.neo.life

Printed in the United States
10 9 8 7 6 5 4 3 2 1

Design: Morla Design, Inc.

Previous spread: An artist's rendering of tissue factor pathway inhibitor,
a molecule that interrupts the process of blood coagulation.

Road Maps

Creative Briefs

Dreams

Introduction

Humans now have the tools to intervene in our own evolution and build a better world. So what should we do with these powers?

We're obsessed with that question. And in the pages that follow, scientists, artists, writers, and entrepreneurs take it on too. They envision radically different futures, when people will manipulate their DNA and make organisms to do their bidding—when the very definition of *Homo sapiens* will be up for grabs.

We *Homo sapiens* of 2020 are just starting down this path, adjusting our fertility and longevity, our food and sleep, our hearts and minds. We could go in lots of directions from here, but this book is optimistic about where the journey will lead, even as we'll be creating living technologies that we can't fully control.

This isn't a comprehensive master plan for humanity. Instead it captures an excited and anxious moment when people are peering beyond the vast neobiological frontier. The essays, stories, images, and interviews that follow are meant to help you imagine what the buildout could look like. Some of these pieces are like creative briefs for bioarchitects of the coming decades. Others are rough road maps for possible technologies, or dreams of how things might unfold. You're not going to agree with every point of view, but that's our intention: Try these ideas on and see how they feel.

Why? Because even as we redirect the flow of biological evolution, cultural evolution still moves faster and more assuredly. Changes in our DNA, whether they come from random mutations or from clever gene therapies, will alter the range of possible human outcomes. But culture—including the scenarios we imagine, the stories we tell, our decisions about which technologies to fund or buy—will determine which of our possible futures actually occur.

The idea that it's all up to us is reassuring, inspiring, and daunting. It's also the most human thing imaginable, the gift and legacy of our species, one apparently possessed by no other animal, not even the other hominins that once roamed the Earth. That trait is, simply, the ability to imagine situations that do not yet exist, and then create them.

Jane Metcalfe, NEO.LIFE founder and publisher
Brian Bergstein, NEO.LIFE editor at large

Shown right: A map of RNA molecules made with DNA microscopy, which captures spatial and genetic data.

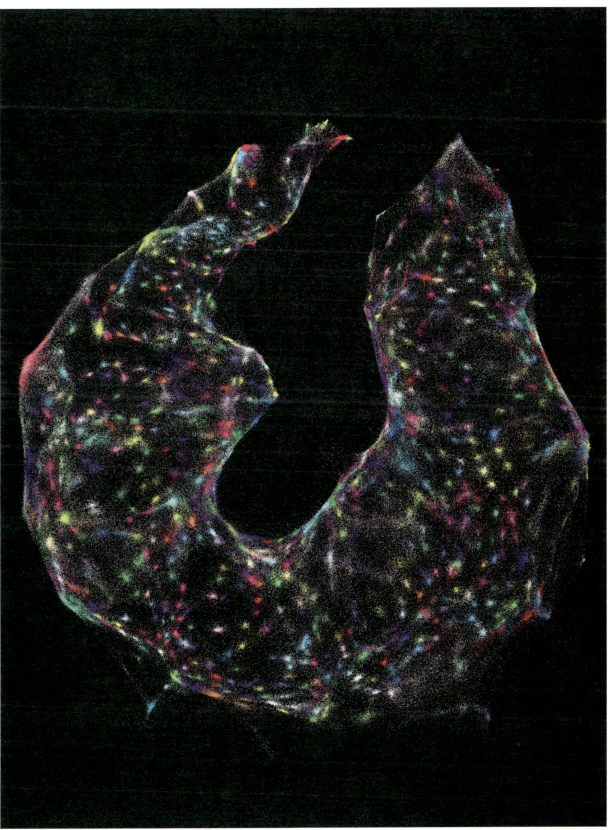

Courtesy of Joshua Weinstein, Broad Institute of MIT and Harvard

Rough Draft of a Manifesto

Jane Metcalfe

Over two days in March 2019, NEO.LIFE convened biologists and other scientists, authors, artists, engineers, entrepreneurs, venture investors, a tech-policy scholar, a roboticist, and a physician (all named in the acknowledgements on page 152) and asked them to come up with plausible scenarios in which biotechnologies dramatically alter the human experience. Then we asked them to consider even bigger questions: What aspects of those scenarios are worth striving for? What values should inform the use of gene editing, synthetic biology, and other fundamental new tools?

Guided by scenario planner Peter Schwartz, the group identified major trends and forces happening right now—everything from increases in the world's population, wealth, and urbanization to climate change and the crisis of democratic governance. Some of us suggested that economic and electronic connectedness will keep international conflicts just short of becoming wars; others pointed to a stultifying absence of meaning and purpose for people in many advanced societies.

We discussed the prospects for space exploration, artificial intelligence, cellular agriculture, artificial gametes, and artificial wombs. We considered the likelihood that biotechnologies can be effectively controlled, and even whether genes and other basic facets of human biology might turn out to be less reliably hackable than many people hope.

What came out of all that? A sense that it's possible to outline a future people can rally for rather than fear. The group articulated these principles:

> Technology should be used to increase biological diversity, both in humans and in other species. This future-proofs our civilization and widens the range of its possibilities.

> In general, people should be free to determine their own use of genetic modification, based on well-informed choices. This framework will help people think about the differing ramifications of, say, a gene therapy on an adult and gene edits on embryos. It also ought to counter claims that biotechnology will unleash a new eugenics.

> As we pursue genetic repairs that cure disease, we should expect that healthy people will use the same tools to enhance their abilities. Rather than parsing whether something amounts to a treatment or an enhancement, it will be far more meaningful to consider whether interventions a) give individuals traits that already have existed in some humans or b) give them entirely new traits that have not arisen before.

> Humility and caution will lower the risk of unintended consequences that would undermine biotechnologies and thus reduce human possibility in the long run. This could mean, for example, that society requires gene edits to always be tested first in somatic cells rather than in the germ line, even if the latter step were technically easier or more efficacious. It should motivate the development of mute switches or other mechanisms for undoing gene edits.

> Governance of biotechnologies should exhibit traits of the underlying system. Biology itself does not recognize strict boundaries; it also reveals the importance of adaptations, feedback loops, and the interplay of ecosystems. It's worth asking whether we can develop regulatory systems that take on such features as well.

Maybe we need a manifesto for the future of *Homo sapiens*. There is much to gain from the effort, but only if everyone weighs in. The handful of principles outlined above are just the start. We're putting them out there now to provoke conversations across disciplines, cultures, geographies, and time.

Let the debate begin.

"It comes up in a lot of bioethical discussions that we should avoid doing things until you're sure that they're safe. I think that's the most risky way of proceeding. What you really want to do to reduce the big risks is to maximize the information flow and fail fast."

GREGORY STOCK | BIOETHICIST

George Church
Ramez Naam

How to Turn Science Fiction into Science Fact

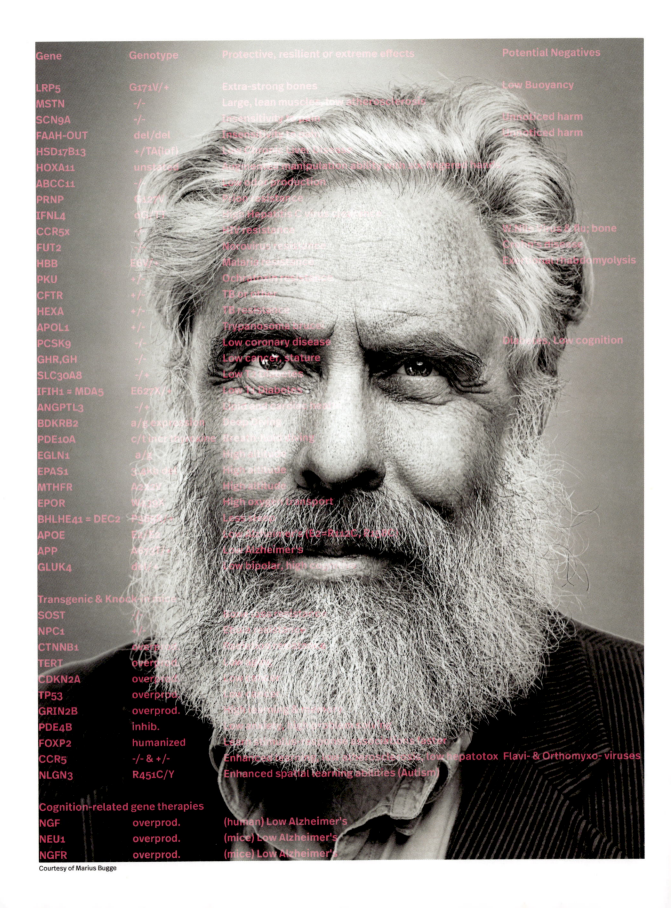

Gene	Genotype	Protective, resilient or extreme effects	Potential Negatives
LRP5	G171V/+	Extra-strong bones	Low Buoyancy
MSTN	-/-	Large, lean muscles, low atherosclerosis	
SCN9A	-/-	Insensitivity to pain	Unnoticed harm
FAAH-OUT	del/del	Insensitivity to pain	Unnoticed harm
HSD17B13	+/TA(lof)	Low chronic liver disease	
HOXA11	unstated	Enhanced manipulation ability with six-fingered hands	
ABCC11	-/-	Low odor production	
PRNP	G127V	Prion resistance	
IFNL4	dG/TT	Slow Hepatitis C virus clearance	
CCR5x		HIV resistance	W.Nile virus & flu; bone
FUT2	-/-	Norovirus resistance	Crohns disease
HBB	E6V/+	Malaria resistance	Exertional rhabdomyolysis
PKU	+/-	Ochratoxin resistance	
CFTR	+/-	TB or small	
HEXA	+/-	TB resistance	
APOL1	+/-	Trypanosoma brucei	
PCSK9	-/-	Low coronary disease	Diabetes, Low cognition
GHR,GH	-/-	Low cancer, stature	
SLC30A8	-/+	Low T2 Diabetes	
IFIH1 = MDA5	E627X/+	Low T1 Diabetes	
ANGPTL3	-/+	Balanced cardiac function	
BDKRB2	a/g expression	deep diving	
PDE10A	c/t intermediate	breath-hold diving	
EGLN1	a/a	High altitude	
EPAS1	3-5kb del	High altitude	
MTHFR	A222V	High altitude	
EPOR	N519X	High oxygen transport	
BHLHE41 = DEC2	P385R	Less sleep	
APOE	E2/E2	Low cardio risks (E2=R112C, R158C)	
APP	A673T/+	Low Alzheimer's	
GLUK4	del/-	Low bipolar, high cog	

Transgenic & Knock-in mice

Gene	Genotype	Protective, resilient or extreme effects	Potential Negatives
SOST		Bone properties	
NPC1	+/-		
CTNNB1	overprod.		
TERT	overprod.		
CDKN2A	overprod.		
TP53	overprod.	Low cancer	
GRIN2B	overprod.		
PDE4B	inhib.		
FOXP2	humanized	Learn stimulus-response associations faster	
CCR5	-/- & +/-	Enhanced cognition, low osteoporosis risk, low hepatotox	Flavi- & Orthomyxo- viruses
NLGN3	R451C/Y	Enhanced spatial learning abilities (Autism)	

Cognition-related gene therapies

Gene	Genotype	Protective, resilient or extreme effects	Potential Negatives
NGF	overprod.	(human) Low Alzheimer's	
NEU1	overprod.	(mice) Low Alzheimer's	
NGFR	overprod.	(mice) Low Alzheimer's	

Courtesy of Marius Bugge

How to Turn Science Fiction into Science Fact

George Church is a geneticist at Harvard Medical School, but that title undersells him. He is very much an engineer, having developed technologies for sequencing DNA, editing genes, and manipulating stem cells. He's also a beguiling prophet of radical biological change who urges caution even as he reminds people how tantalizing it all might be.

Ramez Naam also defies easy categorization. Naam is the chair of energy and environment at Singularity University and author of *More Than Human: Embracing the Promise of Biological Enhancement*, *The Infinite Resource: The Power of Ideas on a Finite Planet*, and the much-admired science-fiction trilogy *Nexus*. Their conversation has been edited for length and clarity.

Ramez Naam: George, you have been less knee-jerk than most people in rejecting ideas that people find pretty far out. When news came from China last year that a scientist had edited the embryos of two girls in an attempt to make them resistant to HIV, there was a wave of condemnation. And you said, "Hold on, let's take a balanced view." Where does that instinct come from?

George Church: Well, it probably comes from doing technology development, including some technology development that's made its way into clinical practice, and seeing the successes and failures in the long history of gene therapy. One thing is to ask what the long-term consequence is going to be: Is it actually likely these kids are going to die, as some people did in the early days of gene therapy?[1]

I've seen things change extremely rapidly. The other part of what's unbalanced in the discussion [of genetics research] is that sometimes people say, "Oh, this stuff is so far off and so impractical, so unlikely, we don't need to really take it seriously." That doesn't prepare us well for a sudden change in technology. For example, bringing down the cost of sequencing from $3 billion for a poor, non-clinical genome, to nearly zero dollars now for a high-quality diploid genome[2], was supposed to take six decades, and instead it took on the order of six to eight years.

You need to discuss the scenarios because a false positive—where you talk about a scenario that never happens—isn't so bad. But a false negative—where you miss a revolution and then end up being reactive rather than proactive—is worse.

---

[1] The HIV resistance gene that scientist He Jiankui tried to edit into the embryos also appears to raise the risk of death from the flu and West Nile virus. Asked to address that, Church responded that the tradeoff might be worthwhile for people in places where HIV poses a bigger threat than the flu.

[2] A diploid genome includes both sets of chromosomes. Early sequencing projects generated composite genomes out of haploid sequences—just one set of chromosomes—from multiple donors.

Shown left: Portrait of George Church overlaid with his list of protective alleles.

Naam: You mentioned an almost-free, high-quality diploid human genome. What's the implication of that?

Church: We've got the infrastructure in place to sequence everybody's genome on the planet. But there's got to be a social revolution and maybe some marketing—just the right combination that will cause us to go past the tipping point. I think it could happen any minute now, and it could immediately save trillions of dollars just with Mendelian diseases alone. We don't even have to discover the basis of complex diseases and all the rest that people think is far off. Just getting the wheels turning on Mendelian diseases and getting that out to everybody equitably could completely change poverty, in industrialized nations as well.

Naam: By Mendelian diseases, you mean diseases that are caused by just one gene?

Church: It could be one or two. Simple diseases that are highly predictive and very serious. They don't have to be curable, but you can fix them. This has been proven with matchmaking, which is very low-cost and doesn't require FDA approval. That's a radical but proven and very inexpensive approach to eliminating some of those serious diseases, often heart-rending family situations.

14

Naam: Just by letting people know what they carry and what their potential mate carries, we can avoid a lot of those?

Church: That's the way it's currently done. But you could do it without anybody knowing that they're carriers. We're all carriers of something. So what you do is, you just get a list of a large number of people who are geographically convenient, in places that you go, who are compatible with you in age, and interest, and genes. That way, you never have to have the heart-rending problem of saying, "Here are two people who are in love" and then they learn they're incompatible, and then they split up. Everybody knows they split up because they're both carriers. That's unnecessary emotional harm and stigmatization.

Naam: I can see the movie script writing itself. It would be a dystopian state that does this matchmaking service. It'd be *Gattaca* meets *Romeo and Juliet*, with gene-crossed lovers who want to be together despite their genetic incompatibility.

Church: No, the thing is, do it as early as possible so that anybody you're thinking seriously about even dating is already on your list. You're not excluding that many people. It's like 5% of the possible dates you'd be excluding. It's not a big–

Naam: Yeah. I mention that movie sort of tongue-in-cheek because society has this tendency to pick not-super-plausible scenarios of harm or damage for new technologies like this and fixate on them, rather than the upsides.

Church: Well, it's not necessarily all bad. Again, the consequences of having a false positive, where we get all worked up about something that doesn't materialize, like Y2K for example, that's not so bad. It's much better than having it sneak up on us and we just weren't ready for it. There are a few internet things that we weren't quite expecting. I think it's better to have the negative scenarios out there. It's all about balance.

Naam: You've compared the Chinese kids who had been gene edited to Louise Brown, the first baby born through in-vitro fertilization. We used to say kids born through IVF were "test tube babies."

Church: Right.

Naam: Do you think 20, 30, 40 years from now it will be the same way with gene-edited human babies? That it'll just have become normalized?

Church: It's quite possible. But there are alternatives. One that we have talked about already is matchmaking. That solves a lot of things. If you had that working, you wouldn't need gene therapies in adults or embryos. Or if male or female infertility can't be fixed by in-vitro fertilization—and there are quite a few that can't—then by definition [gene edits on those people] would be restoring the germ line to an ancestral, healthy, functional state. I think that's an example of something which would be considered as medical as in-vitro fertilization and might be accepted.

Naam: What about people who want to augment? What if somebody wants to have a child and says, "I am heavy and my spouse is heavy, I want them to be a good-looking, normal-weight person." They will justify it as lowering the risk of diabetes, but really it's an aesthetic thing; it's an enhancement. People will want to do that, right?

Church: Yeah. I think that the people that have a particular disease are in the best position to determine whether their children can handle it or not. People who've never had it in their family are not in a good position to judge. I don't think lack of obesity is necessarily going to be considered by everybody to be an enhancement. But there are examples of enhancement that we already have in most industrialized nations, like the immunity to 20 different infectious diseases. We're differentiated from our ancestors. Our ancestors lived in mortal fear of these diseases. We don't. We're also augmented in non-biological ways that have biological impact. For example, if you said, "Well, I'm going to engineer my muscles so I can run really fast." How is that different from hopping in an Uber?

Naam: It's still not as fast as Uber.

Church: Right. Or a jet. Or a rocket. So these days, the need for physical augmentation, biologically, is less than it used to be. We still want to augment, but it's usually through physics and chemistry. There's a strange exceptionalism where we can get augmented one way but not another. We can get augmented as an adult, but not as a baby. There's a lot of lip service to preventative medicine, which could be considered augmentation.

Naam: I'll offer an intellectual augmentation: literacy. Learning to read at an early age rewires the brain biologically.

Church: Perfect example.

Naam: But no one thinks of it because it's baseline now. Are you saying we should be comfortable with offering some of these augmentations in the embryo?

Church: I think it's case by case. My guess is a lot of the augmentation is going to happen in adults first. There are only 100 million babies born each year worldwide, and there are 7.5 billion adults, so it's a bigger market. Also, some of the augmentations will be intrinsically easier to do in adults. Our aging society is going to get us hyper aware of cognitive decline, so we'll want to compensate with cognitive enhancement. It's going to be very hard to resist that possibility. Even though we say that intelligence is incredibly complicated, well, there are plenty of examples of one or two or three genes causing great enhancements of one or many cognitive abilities. It's been shown in animals. Many of these things are candidates for gene therapy in people who have the first symptoms of Alzheimer's or just have some risk for it. Gene therapies in the pipeline today are going in that direction, reducing the probability of cognitive decline in Alzheimer's and other sources of decline. Some of those could result in cognitive enhancement if used by someone who's not in decline.

Naam: Would that be better for society, if we had more people who were smarter?

Church: We need to be cautious. We have to ask, "Are we maintaining the neurodiversity we need?" Autistics have historically been described as intellectually disabled. But very often, if they can become high-functioning, they're the opposite. They contribute things to society that nobody else sees. Same thing could happen with a whole variety of neuro-diversity.

Naam: You have narcolepsy, right?

Church: Yeah. I'm narcoleptic, and when I was young, dyslexic. I have little bits of OCD, as many of my colleagues do.

Naam: So you'd consider yourself neurodiverse?

Church: I would think that I would be one of the ones that you would get rid of if you were trying to squeeze the bell curve down.

Naam: Do you consider any of your neurodiversity a contributing factor for your success?

Church: My gut tells me that I have benefited, that it's been a net positive. Just being different at all from the middle of the bell curve gives you an advantage in a part of society that cherishes innovation and out-of-the-box thinking. That's a part that I managed to find. But I'm sure there are many professions, and different eras, and maybe even different geographies where I would be dead or at least penniless.

Naam: It's interesting because there are all these articles about people in Silicon Valley micro-dosing psychedelics or whatnot, and it almost reads like these people are trying to make themselves temporarily more neurodiverse.

Church: They were born in the middle of the bell curve, and they're trying to escape.

Naam: Could I do that via genetic methods? I read long ago that one of the alleles[3] that has the highest correlation with changes in IQ has an association with higher risk of schizophrenia. What if I want to make myself smarter in some way that might come with other side effects? If I'm an adult, should society allow me to do so?

Church: Well, "shoulds" are difficult. The "should" is: Should society allow you to do that in order for society to achieve a goal like having better books? Or better technologies? I think society could tolerate a few more out-of-the-box thinkers. So it's really a matter of, "Are you endangering yourself to such an extent that you've become a burden on society, where government has to pay for your medical expenses for the rest of your life?"

---

[3] A variation in the letters of a gene.

If that results in you becoming a quadriplegic, society doesn't want that to happen to you, reasonably. The same thing could happen with becoming neurodiverse. I think that something you can turn on and off has a particular attraction over something that's permanent, something that you did in the germ line. Wouldn't it be kind of cool if you got one of my disabilities or autism and could be able to turn it off when you need to be sociable or need to relax or something? Then crank it all the way up when you want to be creative, or have a deadline or something?

Naam: In the field of brain-computer interfaces there are people who talk about using transcranial magnetic stimulation to temporarily induce savant states. I'm not sure anybody really knows if it works or not.

Church: I tend to think it's wishful thinking that there's something you could eat or drink or some convenient thing to put on your head, whether it's infrared or magnetic. When we talk about gene therapy, we would literally have complete access to the whole biological spectrum. All the shortcuts and simple therapies we think of today are going to seem fairly pathetic.

Naam: When we talk about the whole biological spectrum, you're not just talking about genes or alleles that exist in humans today. You're talking about going beyond that, like genes from other species, or genes that just don't exist at all, potentially.

Church: That's right. We need to take that sort of possibility very seriously.

Naam: You've said that the human future in space depends upon editing our genes.

Church: It may not even be considered augmentation. If we're desperately sick due to radiation and low gravity over long periods of time, then that would be considered a medical emergency. It might be acceptable. I do think that there are new challenges that we're already facing in cities that our ancestors weren't fully evolved for, but we'll definitely be facing it in longer-term colonization efforts in space.

Naam: How might we modify ourselves to thrive in space?

Church: Radiation resistance is actually quite well understood. There are some extraordinarily radiation-resistant biological systems that we could move over into human cells, at a minimum. There are problems with osteoporosis and other distribution of fluids in your body that happen at anything less than one unit of gravity. Some of the solutions to that could be used on Earth for osteoporosis, but some of them would be unique. I think we know enough about physiology, or could use our current foundations, to really seriously address those two issues and others. Our microbiomes could be rethought. So could some of the neurobehavioral components of living in close quarters.

Naam: Changing our brains so we're better suited to surviving on a small spaceship or in a small-quarters Mars colony for a very long period of time—what would those changes look like?

Church: Oh, I don't think that the final list of genes is in. We have a short list of genes for longevity and aging reversal, from many animal studies. Some of those will be relevant. We have a short list of cognitive- and anxiety-related genes that have been shown in animal studies as well. One or two or three genes will have a large effect, even though you know there are thousands of genes involved in natural populations. With synthetic biology, you're not limited to the exact alleles or allele frequencies in the natural population.

For osteoporosis, the pathways are understood for osteoplast formation, the cells that build up and break down bones. The genes involved in calcium, metabolism, vitamin D— these are understood. With a little trial and error, we could get it so that animals are not suffering from bone loss. In terms of the fluid distribution, that I know less about, but I'm fairly sure that could be compensated as well.

Naam: You've mentioned longevity. How can we affect the human life span and health span through genetics?

Church: A lot of what makes young cells young is their commitment to doing repair at a good clip. There are 300 genes in Pedro de Magalhães's GenAge database[4] that are up for grabs, and we're looking at a fair number of them in the gene therapy context, so they can be applied to older animals and older people. A huge fraction of what we're going to die from in industrialized nations are diseases that don't kill 20-year-olds. Probably 90% of us will die of such age-related diseases. And if you get some gene therapies that get multiple ones at once, then you're probably on the right track for something that's dealing with the fundamentals of aging rather than just alleviating symptoms. We know the nine pathways of aging[5], and there might be some relatively small numbers of genes that are highly leveraged in those nine pathways. So you just convince the cells that they're younger, and they need to repair. You don't necessarily micromanage the repair, you just convince the cell to do its job.

[4] João Pedro de Magalhães of the University of Liverpool leads a collaborative effort called Human Aging Genomic Resources, which includes GenAge, a database of genes that are known to play roles in aging.

[5] A 2013 paper in *Cell* said nine "hallmarks of aging" are "genomic instability, telomere attrition, epigenetic alterations, loss of proteostasis, deregulated nutrient-sensing, mitochondrial dysfunction, cellular senescence, stem cell exhaustion, and altered intercellular communication."

Naam: Let's go back to the slightly more far out. You made this comment recently: "The human brain may not be at the ideal size." Can you elaborate on that?

Church: It's unlikely that any aspect of our bodies or ecosystems or the environment is fully optimal. The lesson of evolution is that there's constantly room for improvement. In the evolutionary sense, whatever it was that they were trying to do was to maximize procreation. There's a whole new set of criteria that we have today. A lot of the maximized procreation of the past assumed that food was an extremely limited resource. Hence, energy had to be conserved, so you wouldn't waste energy on things like repair, especially after you reproduced. We can reoptimize these systems. Now, back to the brain. If we did start doing adult augmentation, there might be a desire to have a more flexible brain size, just to put new components in. It's not to say that brain size correlates with anything desirable, it's just that, in the transition time, you might say, "Let's just make it bigger." For a while, we made computers a lot bigger. Now, smaller computers are more desirable. But during transition times, you're just very pragmatic about it. I don't know what the right size is but I think functionality will dictate it.

Naam: If you wanted to add functionality to your brain, what kind of upgrades would you be seeking?

Church: I don't think eliminating sleep, though some people put that on their list. I don't think that's necessarily a plus. I think what I would like is more working memory. The lesson we get from computers is the more things you can keep in RAM or even faster parts of the memory, those are advantageous.

Naam: Hold more concepts at once in your mind.

Church: Right. Right now, we see everything in two dimensions, we translate it into three dimensions. We can mathematically talk about four dimensions, but what if that were something that we could more deeply feel? I think that would be more interesting. We talk about consciousness, different levels of consciousness. I know late in the day I feel semi-nonfunctional. What if my very best part of the day was just my average, and then there's something beyond that? Caring for other people: it would be nice to be able to crank that up without necessarily putting one at risk for people who don't care about you.

The list could go on and on. I'm sure that if you get a lot of creative people around the world thinking about this, they will come up with cool ideas and also what's wrong with those cool ideas, how to fix what's wrong with those cool ideas, et cetera. That's why we need a culture of science fiction coupled with a culture of turning science fiction into science fact.

Naam: Speaking of which: You've got an idea for sending small amounts of biological machinery ahead of us to explore or help colonize faraway worlds in space.

Church: Right. It's very difficult right now to get even reasonable-sized electronic probes going at relativistic speeds[6]. If we go at current rocket speeds, even with gravitational assistance, it's going to take us millennia to get to some reasonable place outside of our solar system. So, you really want a strategy by which we could go as close to the speed of light as possible. Obviously, light goes at the speed of light. And if we had a 3D printer at the other end, in principle, we could transmit something to it with copies of ourselves. We're a bit away from making copies of ourselves. But how would you get that 3D printer at the other end, assuming there is nobody else in the universe? Until we find out there's somebody there, we need to put our own printer up there.

What's the smallest package that we could get going at some high fraction of the speed of light? There's been discussion of breakthrough star shots: getting a one-gram package to do a fly-by of one of our nearest solar systems. I think a fly-by will not be that informative. What we really want is to land. And we don't want to send a gram. We want to send a lot less than that, because if a gram hits an atmosphere at relativistic speeds, you have something that's likely the equivalent of an atom bomb. But a nanogram is something that could, conceivably, get accelerated easily and even decelerated at the other end.

There are challenges, definitely, but a nanogram is about the size of a eukaryotic cell. We know that a eukaryotic cell, a single cell, can contain enough information to create a very complex body. For that matter, a population of bodies. It could be programmed with enough information to build a light source that could beam back, bidirectionally, establish a communication line. Then you could start moving things at the speed of light. Not matter, but information.

Naam: I love this. We send a single cell to a faraway world that would self-replicate and build a transmitter and computational strata of some sort there as our first steps to that new world.

Church: Yeah. I think that's the smallest package that we can get going at the highest speed. Maybe even within our lifetime.

---

[6] Einstein teaches us that relativity always applies. Here Church is talking about a sizable fraction of the speed of light.

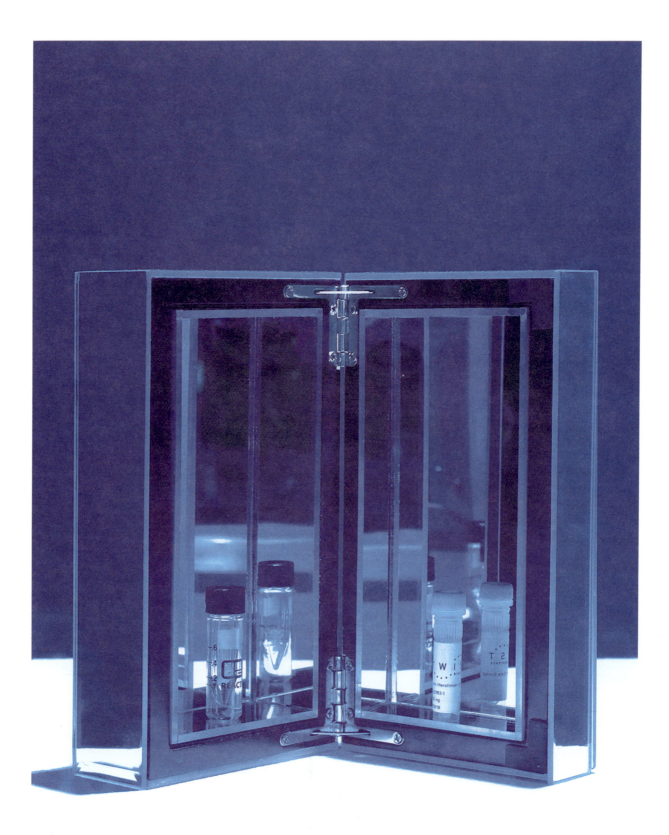

Lynn Hershman
Leeson
Anti-Bodies

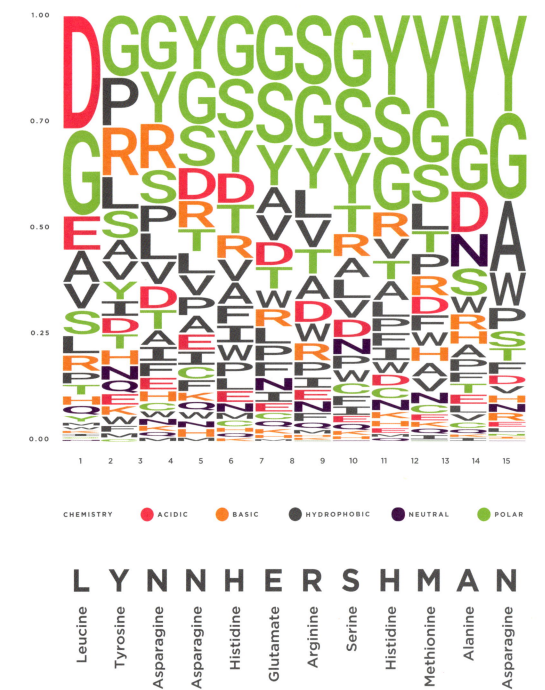

PROBABILITY

CHEMISTRY ● ACIDIC ● BASIC ● HYDROPHOBIC ● NEUTRAL ● POLAR

L Y N N N H E R S H M A N

- Leucine
- Tyrosine
- Asparagine
- Asparagine
- Histidine
- Glutamate
- Arginine
- Serine
- Histidine
- Methionine
- Alanine
- Asparagine

Anti-Bodies

Lynn Hershman Leeson is a San Francisco-based artist and filmmaker who has been at the forefront of using digital and biological technologies for the past 50 years. She celebrates the democratization of technology, but provokes us to think about how we let it define and dominate us. An indignant feminist and a sly jokester, Hershman Leeson delights in pushing new technology in unreasonable ways and uncomfortable directions. Much of her work grapples with identity in an age of bioengineering, pervasive surveillance, and persistent discrimination.

The works on these pages speak directly to our new god-like powers. They are the result of a collaboration with the Swiss pharmaceutical giant Novartis, which led to an exhibition called *Anti-Bodies*. The research scientists generated two antibodies—one based on her name and another called ERTA, named for Roberta Breitmore, a fictional alter ego who has figured frequently in the artist's work.

There are 22 natural amino acids, and DNA tells cells which ones to use in proteins. Both of these fabricated antibodies correspond to the string of amino acids spelled out by her name L (leucine) Y (tyrosine) N (asparagine) H (histidine) E (glutamic acid) R (arginine) S (serine) H (histidine) M (methionine) A (alanine) N (asparagine). The LYNNHERSHMAN antibody is capable of binding to a broad variety of proteins, much like its socially active namesake. The fictitious character Roberta Breitmore's antibody cannot bind to any known proteins, so neither would have any therapeutic value.

Of the two vials featured on page 22, one contains an archive of the artist's work—including documents, photos, and films—stored in DNA, thanks to the synthetic biology company Twist Bioscience. The second vial contains the powder essence of the LYNNHERSHMAN antibody. Together these vials suggest eternal preservation for both the artist and her work, and the possibility of reviving one or both in the ultimate artistic comeback. Although someone still needs to invent a way to play back the film from DNA.

Previous spread: Detail of "Room #8": LYNNHERSHMAN and ERTA antibodies, DNA, mirror box, lab door. Created in collaboration with Novartis and HeK, House of Electronic Arts Basel. Size variable, edition of four, collection of ZKM Museum, 2007-2018.

Shown left: In a paper published about the project, Novartis scientists illustrate the chances of the LYNNHERSHMAN antibody existing in nature. Each of the vertical lists of letters above her name are arranged to indicate the likelihood that any given amino acid would be found in that position in the sequence of naturally generated human antibodies. The larger the letter, the more often that particular amino acid tends to occur at that place in an antibody sequence.

Next spread: Lynn Hershman Leeson with the LYNNHERSHMAN antibody.

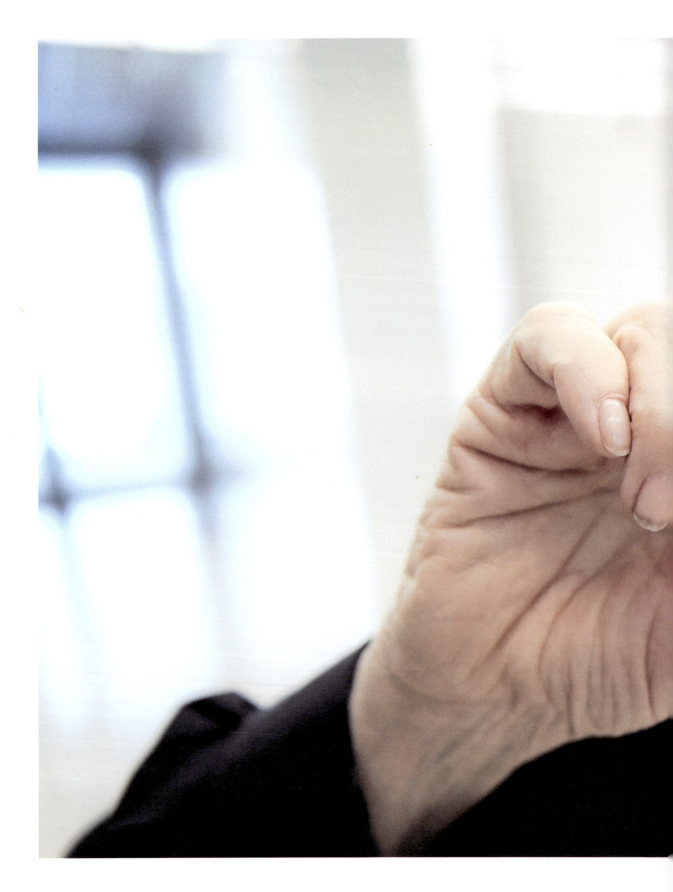

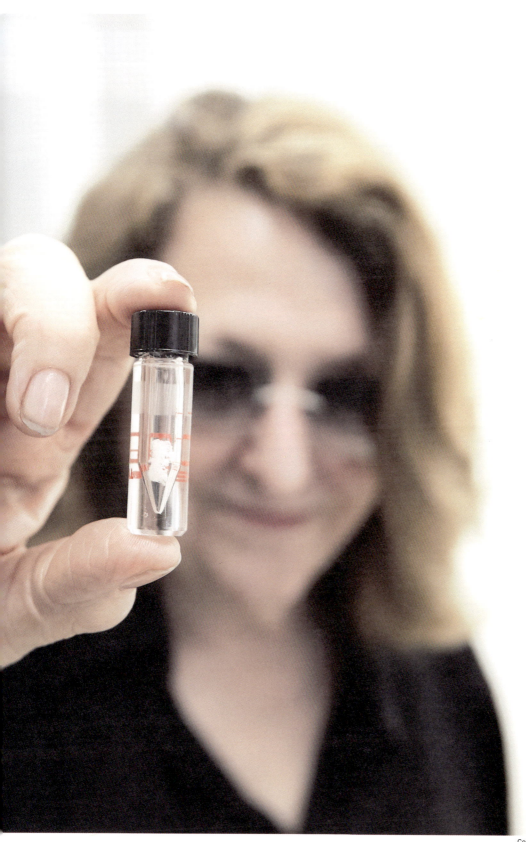

"We don't want a world that's perfect, because if we do—
and we're headed towards that world—we're all going to
look the same."
LUCY MCRAE | ARTIST

Nicola Patron

Botanists Could Save Us All

Botanists Could Save Us All

Nicola Patron leads a synthetic biology research group at the Earlham Institute, a life-sciences center in Norwich, England. Her lab is engineering photosynthetic organisms that can churn out valuable molecules used in medicine and agriculture. Her team also investigates ways to make food crops that are healthier and require fewer chemicals.

The word "botanist" conjures images of pith-helmeted plant-collectors waist-deep in the tangled vines of tropical jungles, but this is not what I do. I'm at the interface of plant biology and engineering, and much of my work is focused on human health and nutrition. Botanists hold not only seeds but the very future of the human race in our slightly dirty hands.

Even some highly respected scientists are alarmingly oblivious of our work. A few years ago I joined an effort to examine how large bioresources, such as DNA databases and tissue banks, could spark transformative research. An eminent clinician was puzzled as to why a botanist was invited to comment at all. I explained that having access to plant tissues, seeds, and DNA sequence information is essential for studying and improving, among other things, yield and nutrition in crops. I emphasized how critical this work is for food security and for preventing undernutrition, which causes 45% of all deaths among children younger than 5. He said he'd never thought about botany—or botanists— in that way.

There is no Nobel Prize for plant science. Norman Borlaug is estimated to have saved a billion human lives by using science to improve agriculture, and in 1970 they gave him the Nobel Peace Prize. Perhaps this is not unfitting; spikes in food prices after crop failures frequently lead to political and social unrest.

The world's population has swelled by about 5 billion since Borlaug's Green Revolution, and feeding the population of 2050 will require a 40 to 70% increase in farm production. Averting this potential crisis by turning more land over to farming would be disastrous. We need to keep every remaining forest, wetland, and grassland and rewild degraded lands. While efforts to improve farming practices and reduce food waste are essential, these will not be enough.

Meanwhile, alternative foods produced with new technologies may fuel gastronomic trends in rich countries, but they are unlikely to be relevant or affordable for people in the most food-insecure regions. And reverting to older and less-productive crop varieties and farming practices is not a viable option. Changing all of the world's farms so that they meet the current definition of organic would require an extraordinary amount of extra land–anywhere from 40% to 100% more–to feed even our current population.

It's clear that food security and sustainable agriculture depend on our ability to improve the genetics of crops. Fortunately, we are developing ways to do this with more speed and precision than ever before.

Plants are not defenseless organisms, submissively storing carbon until they are felled by wild weather, herbivores, or combine harvesters. They deal with pests, environmental threats, and even the loss of entire organs by deploying an extensive molecular armory. At school, kids learn that plants respond to light. They can watch plants modulate their direction of growth; perhaps they also visualize how the plants store carbohydrates in preparation for darkness. What the schoolkids can't see is how plants immediately and continually respond to changes such as the availability of nutrients or the presence of pathogens by altering the expression of *thousands* of genes. For example, when the availability of nitrogen shifts even slightly, a plant might adjust the dials for genes that control the length and branching of roots, the rate of growth, and when to produce flowers.

New computational techniques are helping to identify exactly how these changes are coordinated. At the same time, our ability to make purposeful changes to DNA is advancing in leaps and bounds. While older technologies allowed rather crude and random insertions of new genes, molecular tools such as CRISPR let scientists delete, rewrite, or insert sequence information at specific locations.

Now we can test hypotheses about the function of specific sequences and produce plants that don't contain foreign genetic material but have, for example, healthier carbohydrate profiles: rather than causing spikes in blood sugar, they nourish gut microbiota. My lab is exploring how tiny changes to certain DNA sequences, even single letters, can alter plants' responses to environmental signals. We then try to engineer plants to maintain high yields with fewer chemical fertilizers, even in suboptimal environments. Other groups are identifying the genes involved in disease resistance and re-coding them to protect against wider ranges of pathogens. Plants thus equipped would require far fewer applications of chemical control agents.

People have been changing the content and combinations of the genes in crop plants for millennia. Traditional breeding and mutation technologies make thousands of unpredictable changes to plant genes, meaning that improved varieties take years, even decades, to develop. In contrast, biotechnology allows botanical engineers to unlock biodiversity lost through millennia of inbreeding and to collect the most beneficial combinations of genetic variants in a single variety.

These small changes are equivalent to the genetic mutations that produce the natural variations between individuals that are essential for the adaptation and survival of every species. Indeed, many of the sequences we have engineered probably exist in another plant somewhere on the planet. Until now, the challenge has been to identify the genetic variations that are useful and to bring them into high-yielding plant varieties with the speed necessary for farming in a changing climate and for a rapidly expanding population. A new generation of genomics is making this possible.

Botanists may be plant collectors, but we are also ethicists, geneticists, biochemists, and molecular biologists who are trying to create crops that are healthier and have less environmental impact.

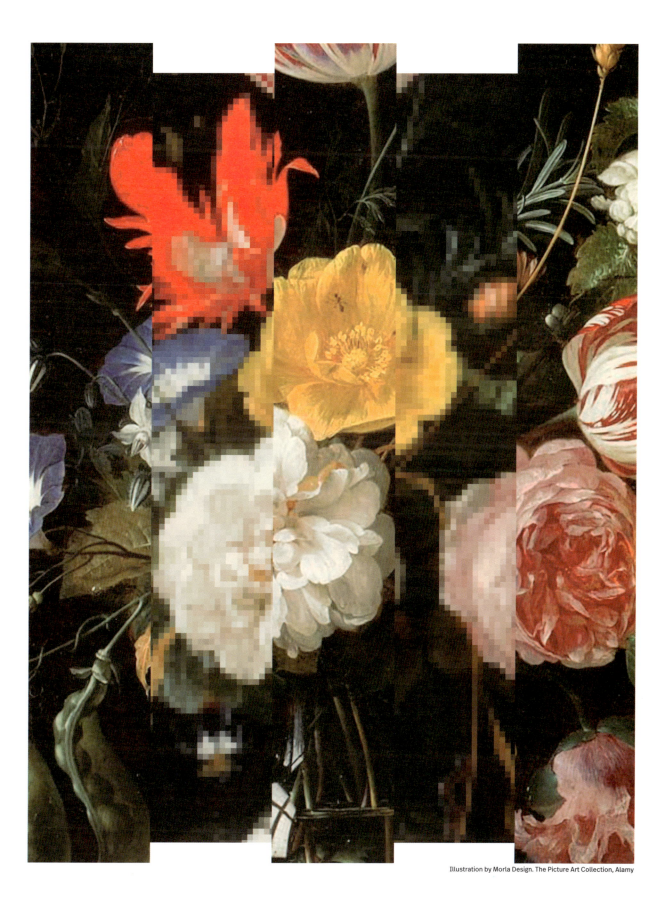

"For countless generations we believed we were special, but science has shown us that we are only as special as everything else. Is this a paradox? Maybe not. Maybe stripping away the delusion of power is the most empowering thing of all."
ELIOT PEPER | SCIENCE-FICTION AUTHOR

Seth Bannon

Us and the Other Animals

Us and the Other Animals

Seth Bannon is a founding partner at Fifty Years, a venture capital firm that focuses on technologies meant to solve big problems. The firm gets its name from a 1931 essay in which Winston Churchill predicted nuclear power, genetic engineering, cultured meat, and other technologies that are still emerging.

A few things might converge in an interesting way.

One is cellular agriculture. Today we functionally use animals as technologies to convert plant proteins into outputs that we like to eat, drink, or wear. There's a new crop of technologies that are just using biology directly to make those things. So our reliance economically and even socially on animals might diminish entirely, and we might not need to use them to live the lives we want to lead.

Two, there's a secular trend in the research of animal cognition where the more we learn, the more we realize they're far more intelligent than we thought before, and they have far more complex social structures and far more complex emotional lives.

Three, we are on the cusp, many people believe, of generating our own intelligence in silicon that may, in the next 50-100 years, put us to shame in terms of its raw intelligence. I think it will cause us to come to grips with the fact that pure intelligence is not the metric by which we should determine how we treat different species of animals.

And then, finally, if the ability to engineer biology is really democratized, you can imagine people doing all sorts of weird things that make animals smarter, or more compassionate, or who knows what. We do that already, through the very slow process of animal breeding, but the speed may increase drastically with genetic engineering techniques.

All these things might come together to radically redefine *Homo sapiens*' relationship with non-human animals.

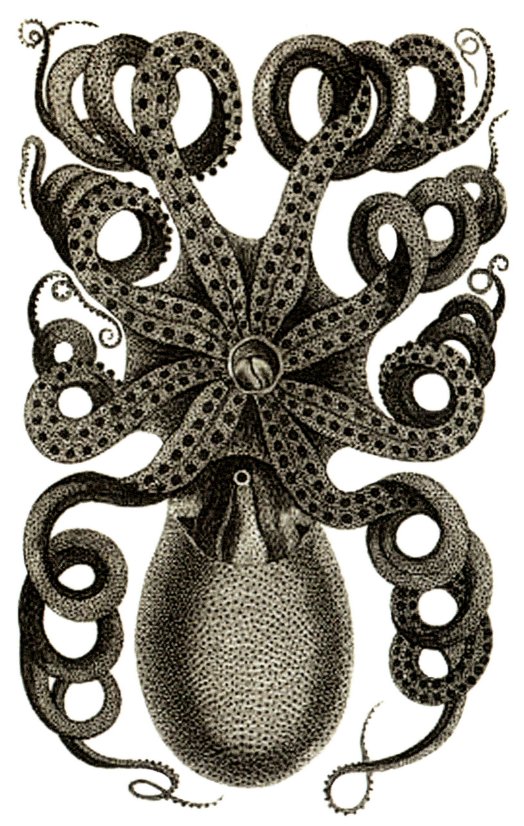

"If you're an adult, and of sound mind, and want to modify yourself, there's very little that society can do to put a stop to that. So, if you wanted to add a tail or glow in the dark, or modify your eyes even, then tech is coming soon and I would not stand in your way."

ANDREW HESSEL | CO-EXECUTIVE DIRECTOR | GP-WRITE

Danny Hillis

Six Things to Think About When Designing Your Child

Six Things to Think About When Designing Your Child

Danny Hillis, inventor and entrepreneur, founded Thinking Machines, a maker of supercomputers; Applied Minds, a technology R&D think tank; and Applied Invention, which develops technologies for companies in agriculture, transportation, manufacturing, energy, medicine, and other fields. He is a cofounder of the Long Now Foundation.

Congratulations on your decision to procreate! This is a short guide to some questions that you should consider before meeting with your genetic architect. If you intend to combine your genetic material with others, we encourage you to discuss these questions with any co-parents in advance.

Everyone wants their descendants to be healthy and happy, but how is that best achieved? When designing your child, keep in mind that you are designing not just an individual, but a member of society. Consider in particular how the child will relate to you and your family.

Here are some of the first questions you should consider:

Size: While it is possible in principle for children to be a continuum of sizes from miniatures to giants, public infrastructure is optimized to support only the three most common sizes: small, classic, and large. Half-sized children are by far the most economical. These small kids, or "demis," consume less than one quarter of the resources of classics. They can live in split-floor housing and take advantage of split-seat transportation. Also, their shorter neurons allow them to think faster. Large children, or "supers," are also a popular choice, especially for parents who value athletic performance. Keep in mind, however, that their advantages in physical power come with greater needs for space and other resources. Supers can also be a challenge to raise, especially for small and classic-sized parents. If you're living in a city with older infrastructure, or if you value a traditional lifestyle, a classic-sized child may still be your best choice.

Additional appendages: While some parents still opt for the traditional pair of five-fingered hands, we recommend that you consider at least one additional appendage. Prehensile tails have pluses and minuses, but there is very little downside to an extra set of fingers or a few small tentacles. Studies have shown that children without these features often wish they had them.

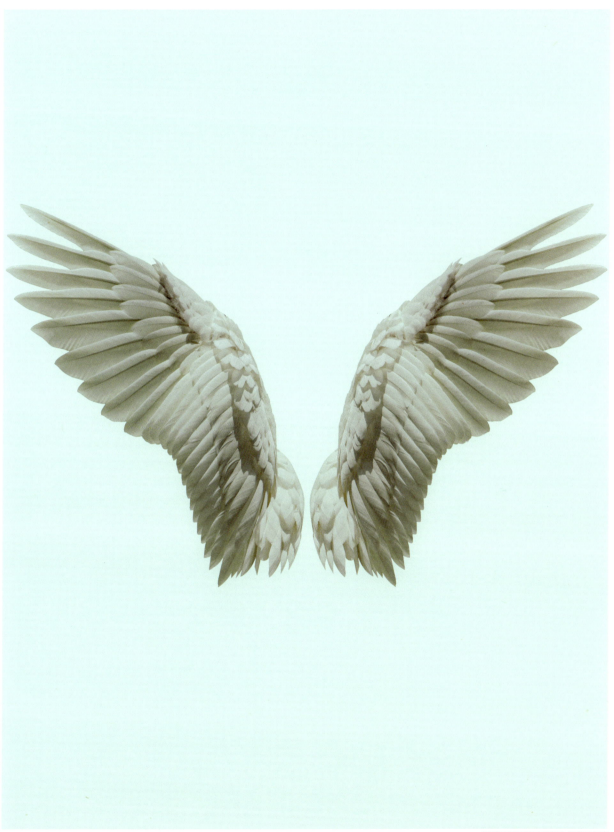

Mental predispositions: Choosing your child's brain type requires some trade-offs. For instance, every parent would like their child to be good at abstract thinking and have high sensory awareness, but these two traits fundamentally compete with each other. The same can be said for emotional and rational intelligence, self-discipline and spontaneity, loyalty and open-mindedness. Our general recommendation is not to push for extremes and strive for a balance. While it is true that people with atypical minds make some of the greatest contributions to science, art, literature, music, and politics, these people are generally not the happiest. If you are concerned that your child will be lonely, consider clones.

Accessories: Wings, tusks, antlers, and trunks are generally not recommended. Extra eyes, redundant internal organs, extended range vision and hearing, cyber interfaces, and extended memory are all worth considering. If you live an aquatic lifestyle, webbing and fins are a must. Gills can extend submersion time, but they are not as useful as extra lung capacity, and they are difficult to keep clean. Echolocation is another popular accessory. The only real limitation to accessorizing is neural bandwidth and metabolic consumption. Your genetic architect will help you find a workable combo.

Gender: Deciding whether to install a Y-chromosome is just the beginning. Contrary to common assumptions, it is not just a matter of picking out primary and secondary sexual characteristics and sexual orientation. You also have a choice of hormone balances and how they vary with time. Sexual preferences, as well as level of sexual interest, can be programmed to change on a monthly cycle. Give some thought to pheromones. It is important that sexual attraction is in sync with sexual attractiveness. And don't underestimate the value of those additional appendages.

Aesthetics: While the exterior covering of a child may seem superficial, the reality is that many parents devote most of their planning to this feature. Fortunately, you have plenty of options for expressing your creativity.

The biggest decision is whether you want to go with a classical pattern of beauty, or something unusual. One popular approach is to select a generally admired form, such as Elf, Prince, or Venus, and customize it with special coloration. Skin pigments are available in all the colors of the rainbow.

Most parents stick to a single hue, using patches of fur, scales, or feathers to add contrasting highlights. Keep in mind, though, that those additions create challenges for thermal control and can be hard to groom.

Patterns such as stripes and spots are possible, but their exact shapes cannot be pro-grammed. Dynamic coloration, or "chameleon effects," can be charming, but will be difficult for your child to control. A good rule of thumb on coloration is to avoid the temptation to follow the latest trend. Those lime and fuchsia stripes on the hottest pop star may look fashionable today, but imagine how your child will feel every time they run into someone their own age, sporting the same pattern. It is generally better to go with coloration that is either traditional or unique. Of course, whatever you do, resign yourself to the fact that most children will seek genetic cosmods when they come of age.

These guidelines are just a starting point for your conversation. Your genetic architect is an expert in helping you design a unique addition to our diverse human society. Remember: Your child's happiness will rest largely on their ability to interact with others and play a positive role in society.

Designing your child is designing the future. Do it wisely.

"I wish for humanity to transition from living on Earth to living with the Earth—for our civilization to be flourishing in partnership with the planet by the time that we're synthesizing human genomes routinely."

DREW ENDY | SYNTHETIC BIOLOGIST

Juan Enriquez

True Human Diversity Is Finally Possible. Will We Be Ready?

True Human Diversity Is Finally Possible. Will We Be Ready?

Juan Enriquez is managing director of Excel Venture Management, which invests in life-science companies. He is an author of four books, most recently *Evolving Ourselves: How Unnatural Selection and Nonrandom Mutation Are Shaping Life on Earth.*

While we humans like to think of ourselves as wildly diverse, any alien coming to Earth and systematically cataloging its life forms would find us singularly boring. There are many, many species and subspecies of birds, bees, bacteria, and cats, but humans are almost identical. The variations between people occur in only 0.1% of our genomes.

This is really odd. Natural selection favors more variation because it provides the ability to adapt to various ecological niches. Variation leads to long-term protection and survival under different circumstances, like plagues and climate change. When you depend on one and only one variant, you can end up in the midst of an Irish potato famine. In strict biological terms there is not nearly enough human diversity.

We have not experienced even small tastes of true diversity for millennia. Although there were once 30-something species of proto-humans, we have not seen or mated with one even mildly different from us for a long time. In fact, we don't actually seem to like the idea of having more human diversity. The notion of making small changes to a fetus elicits horror and revulsion. We probably would be quite uncomfortable living side by side with restored and revived variants of our proto-species. How would you feel about the (literal) Neanderthal dude next door?

But soon we'll need to cope with true diversity within our species. We are not just talking variants of ourselves that *Homo sapiens* could mate with.

The era of space travel, and potentially space colonization, may just force the issue of true speciation. Launch a human body into space and it dramatically decays. Almost all long-term astronauts come back severely damaged by their jaunts, in their vision, hearts, bones, brains. So if we are to leave this place, we are going to have to seriously reengineer the human body, very deliberately, to induce the kind of evolutionary adaptations required for surviving higher radiation, different gravity, more extreme environments. Those engineered humans would be diverse, and the differences between them and humans of today would increase rapidly as successive generations of them got further and further from Earth and adapted to truly different ecosystems.

Even if we do not begin to colonize space in the near future, the human genome will diversify by other means. As more and more gene therapies come online to deal with horrid diseases, the tools necessary for such procedures will become more standardized and widespread. People will use these tools to engineer their own genes and organs, and they won't do it the same way everywhere, especially if different countries adopt different regulations, restrictions, and incentives.

Symbiotic implants may also splinter *Homo sapiens*. Already, engineered limbs are giving athletes abilities beyond those of "normals." Some implants will give people super hearing, in tones we cannot perceive, or super sight. But only some humans will have these powers, especially if the upgrades are expensive.

Historically, when we have encountered perceived human diversity, it has not usually ended well. For millennia, minute variations in skin color, height, or eye shape have justified slavery, serfdom, and other forms of oppression. Everyone knows "that" group is different, and therefore "that group" should be treated differently.

Now we're on the verge of having humans emerge with much bigger differences. True diversity potentially implies different life spans, bodies, and intelligence. Given our very checkered history of how we have treated "others," it is high time to consider the consequences and rules for emerging human variants. We may want to think carefully about the rights and protections we provide to existing species that demonstrate different forms of intelligence, like apes, octopi, dolphins, and whales.

How we treat them and interact may be a blueprint for the customs and laws we will develop as *Homo sapiens* begins to speciate.

"Our goal is to bring more people into the conversation about what's happening in biotech. We have to democratize the technology, and make sure people will have access. We are a movement for social change."

MARIA CHAVEZ | EXECUTIVE DIRECTOR OF BIOCURIOUS

Steve Ramirez

How to Manipulate Memories

How to Manipulate Memories

Steve Ramirez can erase specific memories from mouse brains, reactivate lost memories, and implant false ones. He also is developing ways of tuning memories up or down—enhancing the recollection of positive experiences or quieting negative ones. Ramirez, an assistant professor at Boston University, does this by adding a light-sensitive protein into individual neurons, which makes it possible to activate or deactivate those cells with pulses of light. Although this technique isn't necessarily meant to be used in humans, it's revealing how memory works, which could pave the way for targeted treatments for anxiety, post-traumatic stress disorder, or even Alzheimer's.

NEO.LIFE's editor at large, Brian Bergstein, asked Ramirez to describe how people of the future might think about their pasts.

What are the implications of your work? Where is this all going?
Where the field is really going now is to appreciate that memories are distributed throughout the brain.

When we were tinkering with memories, we would do so by going into a small subregion of the mouse brain and finding cells that held on to a memory. Turning those cells on ended up causing this domino effect, not unlike when you're walking down the street and you catch a glimpse of a cupcake that reminds you of a bake sale from high school. Memories are dynamic. When you recall them, brain cells are firing like crazy. Different areas in the brain start syncing up with one another and start rhythmically communicating with each other. Memories have sights and sounds and smells and emotions, and all of those different modalities recruit different parts of the brain.

With the tools and techniques that are being developed, being able to get a brain-wide image of a single memory is within reach. That's a goal, at least for me, within the next five or 10 years, tops: Can we make a map of either a single memory or two memories? If they're a positive memory and a negative memory, where do they interact? Where do they stop overlapping? We can begin to dynamically map out how the brain cells that hold on to a memory evolve over time.

This research requires implants that shine light into the heads of the mice. Could such an invasive apparatus be used on people?
The brain doesn't have pain receptors, so it's not like it hurts the mice. But we're not going to be sticking optic fibers and microscopes in people's brains. What I'm hoping is that the work that we do in animals provides a kind of blueprint for how the brain might work in a human. So, we can say, "Well, a few areas seem to be key nodes that hold on

to memories." Or, "These areas seem to be those that are deteriorated, for instance, in cases of Alzheimer's" and so on. Then, let's start hunting for that in humans, and see if maybe tools like MRI and so on can find the similar effect or not.

Or, it could go the other way around too, where in humans we can say, "Well, there are certain symptoms of depression where maybe there is discoordinated activity across a handful of brain areas." Now, let's try to create an animal model that mimics that, and then in animals we can figure out what the mechanism is, and then maybe we can make a new drug or a new interventional technique to try to fix the brain, and then translate that idea back to humans. A pill will always be as noninvasive as it gets, because even though we do things like deep brain stimulation in humans, it still is a pretty drastic, last-ditch effort.

Will we someday be able to modify people's experiences of their memories—to dampen the negative ones and enhance the positive ones? And even if it is possible, should we do it?
I would say we're already doing that.

Who are you? Are you the person who is before or after a cup of coffee in the morning? Are you *you* at 7am, are you *you* at 4pm, or are you *you* after two beers at 9pm? We can see already how all the different things that we ingest can change our personalities for instance, and it's the same with memories too. Our memories are not as great if we are sleep-deprived or if we don't do any kind of aerobic work.

In the far future, let's say memory manipulation becomes a thing that you could do at a clinic. For me, one of the ways of using it in a morally responsible way is to keep it in a medicinal setting, keep it in a clinical setting, where you're not just going to go in and erase a memory of a high school breakup just because you don't want to take the two weeks that it's going to take to get over it. You give it to a patient with PTSD and turn the volume down on a traumatic experience. I'm not going to get to enhance a positive memory of the Patriots winning the Super Bowl just because I want to relive it. While that's seemingly fun, you don't know what the side effects would be. But you would do it on a patient with depression, where you can turn the volume up on different aspects of a feeling of motivated positivity and so on. Then I think it can be used in a way that prevents abuse. This is of course the idealist in me talking, but I think that's at least one tractable path forward.

That makes sense if we're talking about dampening specific negative memories or increasing access to positive ones. How should we think about more general potential

upgrades of our memory skills? Let's say there isn't a trauma somebody is trying to get away from; it's just that they want to be better at their job or better at remembering names. What if your work leads to that kind of enhancement?

We know that living a healthy dietary lifestyle, working out, getting a good night's sleep, are all things that could boost your mood, it can boost your memory. All those things are doing something in the brain. So if there was a way to figure out what it's doing to the brain, and then try to artificially reinstate that, like if we could have some kind of drug that mimics the effects of social enrichment or exercise or a good night's sleep or something, then I think that would be awesome. Medicine and our diets and everything around us helped us double our lifespan in the past 200 years. So, maybe this is a way of also doubling what we're cognitively capable of in the next 200 years. But that's just a wild speculation.

The humongous asterisk here is that this is ripe for a million and one different side effects, unless we really knew how to make it that specific in the brain. Right now we're not even close. Any drug that you ingest is going to flood your brain. Caffeine is something that generally makes people wake up and feel a little bit better during the day. But it's not like it's acting on one part of the brain. It'll have its effects of giving you a temporary high or giving you mood-boosting effects, but then, you get things like addiction. Then you get caffeine withdrawal, and you get caffeine-withdrawal-induced migraines and all these things. So, that's the thing: We are playing with a slippery slope here.

What if the military decides to put soldiers into more horrific situations rather than trying to avoid them, knowing that later at the VA hospital they're just going to reduce the sting of the memories or erase them altogether? Could we be setting up a new moral hazard?

There's a pessimistic and optimistic answer. My pessimistic answer is: Let's take something like water, which is the most nurturing thing that we know of. Three quarters of our body, we need it to survive, we drink it every day and so on. But then this thing that nourishes us every day can also be used to waterboard somebody. Something like water can be abused. Now, that doesn't mean that that should be okay. It just means it's a cautionary tale.

With memory manipulation, ideally we use it for the good. A few hundred years from now, hopefully there isn't war. That would be the best solution: don't put people in a traumatic experience to begin with. But let's say it continues. Ideally, should somebody experience something traumatic, then we can use [memory manipulation] for the sake of increasing their well-being, rather than creating somebody who does not experience trauma or who does not perceive of a traumatic situation as traumatic. Because then you end up just making a psychopath.

So, the short answer is yeah, everything can be abused. But I think that one solution is to look at success stories in the past.

In the 1980s, when the Human Genome Project was started, there was a bunch of commentary of "Does this mean we're going to start editing our babies? And then we're going to have this master of race of babies that are genetically modified and all have blonde hair and so on and so forth." That was a couple of decades before the human genome was completed. That commentary has been going on for almost 40 years now. And while it's not perfect we at least now have a social infrastructure that has these problems at the forefront of people's minds.

Ideally that kind of social and legal conversation is what can give us [something like] seat belts to prevent misuse of any technology in this case. I think that's the case with memory manipulation. We surely can think of a million different *Inception-Black Mirror-Total Recall* scenarios where it can be misused. But I'd like to think that through these conversations like the one we're having, at least we can now begin getting this part of the zeitgeist, a social conversation of "Should we?" "What are the pros?" "What are the cons?" So that 40, 50 years from now, when the equivalent of the Human Genome Project in the brain is close to complete, we have an infrastructure in place to prevent misuse. It kind of stinks that it takes that amount of time, because we're working with some very powerful ideas here. But on the other hand it gives us a tractable path forward to make sure it's handled properly.

You make interesting analogies to other technologies, but memory-related technologies scare me more. We are our memories, and it's unsettling to realize they could be made even more fungible. I don't know how to process that. Is it the end of truth?
I don't think it's the end of truth. Truth is an objective data point that simply exists, in my opinion. If anything, this is the beginning of an empowering realization that our memories are indeed malleable and that our recollections can shape-shift just a tad more than we expected. On the cautionary side, it means we need more than eyewitness accounts, for instance. On the uplifting side, we've uncovered something fundamental about what makes us human.

Oshiorenoya Agabi

Future Brains Demand a New Kind of Society

Future Brains Demand a New Kind of Society

Oshiorenoya Agabi is founder and CEO of Koniku, a startup in Berkeley, California, that is developing devices with both electronics and living neurons. Its first product is designed to sniff out dangerous chemicals at airport security. Koniku means "immortal" in Yoruba, a language Agabi learned while growing up in Nigeria.

My medium is neurotechnology. It's the most powerful technology we will ever deploy. It's from there that everything will stream out. Eventually you could use it to modify the duration of life. You could modify the wavelengths people can see. You could add and remove senses. You could design or build awareness or intelligence—whatever that will mean to the people of the future—from scratch. You could combine multiple consciousnesses and you could share them. You could transport consciousness to live in a virtual world for as long as desired.

But it's irresponsible to look at one piece of technology and evangelize it separate from everything else. It leads to a lopsided outcome. If you have such a powerful technology and you deploy it for commercial reasons alone, well, you couldn't design a better dystopia. We can't just say, "Here is this toy, go play with it, and let's make money out of it."

One of the things biotech does is put our own evolution into our hands. Up until now it has all been chance. You can actually have intelligent design now, to put that term to good use. Why should we not radically do the same with society?

Society is shaped for the better when intentional and willing people counteract the harmful disengagement and fear of unwitting players. That is the story of America and the founding fathers who crafted a new society. And today there should be more conversation about how our financial systems and our political systems could be more just. We should be more responsible. Maybe a company should spend half its profits on improving science education. Capitalism is really a great system—it's the best we have, in my view. But we have a "short-termism" problem. That basically means we don't care much about future generations and preserving our species, much less the planet that sustains us. All of us pretend we do, in nice heartwarming words, but in actions we demonstratively do not. I don't know if science or technology will push people to be better, but one way or another, it has to happen.

The first task for technologies that connect any two brains to each other will be to solve the problem of empathy. How do you get two sapiens to fundamentally understand and trust each other? Language is unfortunately inadequate for this: It locks us up in the prison of our minds. We can overcome that with a technology to record from billions of brain cells simultaneously. It would have to be a minimally invasive technology, operating in real time. Additionally or alternatively, we'll need a trusted technology that allows us to process outputs from another person and provides clean and unbiased analysis. But this technology should have none of the middlemen who attach themselves today to less fundamental technologies—speculators and "rent seekers" who create no value and exist solely to generate profit. Such entities shouldn't have access to anyone's brain. This is why we'll need new economic systems that adequately allocate resources and modulate our natural impulses to amass and be selfish.

Our aim with neurotechnology should be to connect and share experiences, to live with another and see the world through others' eyes, to live in one another's skin. On this foundation, for the first time, man would free himself from the deformity that prevents him from standing tall and leaning on the minds of others. Then we would see collectively without hindrance. We would gaze at what really ought to be—traveling within and without.

I believe this thought has always been with man—a state of living and being which our mind, in spite of ourselves, always sensed would be the natural conclusion. But until this age, we have not been able to clearly articulate this collective vision. Now, we have the scientific tools to do so.

The range of applications that could be built on this system or platform (I can't resist the term) is vast. Listing them would require a full book. I hope they are driven not by profit, but by a spirit of curiosity and the need to know ourselves and to live with others.

"I think we've just started to scratch the surface of how
hibernation strategies can be applied to people."
MATT ANDREWS | SLEEP RESEARCHER

David Eagleman

The Children You Could Have Produced Instead

The Children You Could Have Produced Instead

David Eagleman is a neuroscientist and the author of several books, including *Incognito: The Secret Lives of the Brain* and *The Runaway Species.* He is also cofounder and CEO of NeoSensory, a startup developing devices that will extend humans' senses.

Say you have eight frozen embryos. You can use genetic testing to discover what diseases are expected in each embryo, and then select the one with the fewest health risks. This is great news for your child's future. But there's no real reason to stop there: after all, genetic testing grows more discerning each year. Which eye color would you like? How tall is each embryo expected to be? Which one will grow into the most muscular athlete? What will each embryo look like a few decades from now—and why shouldn't you choose the most attractive one? All those options will give us more choice about our children than any previous generation ever dreamt.

That's great, right? Maybe not. Put aside the concern that biological diversity will decrease as certain traits win out; instead, I want to address a psychological point. Parents generally have operated by a simple principle: we get the kids we get. They are the cards we're dealt.

But in the near future, many parents will be able to say "I choose number 5" instead of "I choose number 7." Parental brains will wrestle with questions they have never before faced in reproduction. Their children will share a bedroom with the *what-if* ghosts of the other children that could have taken his or her place.

So while choosing embryos seems like a good move for lowering the disease burden of the next generation, it promises to alter the psychology of parenting. How? Because of what's sometimes called the paradox of choice: the more options you have, the less satisfied you'll be. This has been demonstrated in countless scenarios. Imagine you enter a store that offers dozens of flavors of ice cream. After you've made your choice, you'll enjoy your cone—but it turns out you would have enjoyed the same one even *more* if there were fewer choices, or no choice at all. This same effect is seen in studies from appliances to cars to mates.

Embryo choosing, therefore, offers a new opportunity for regret: a disappointment about active choices we have made ("I'll choose number 3") rather than the single, passive outcome we're used to ("here's your new baby!"). When your child throws a temper tantrum, lying down in the store aisle and kicking the floor, a thought may flit through your consciousness: What if I had chosen embryo number 4 instead? Let's be clear that embryo number 4 would not be free of tantrums. But the brain's capacity to simulate *what ifs* would set you wondering.

Or say you selected embryo 5, believing it was free of genetic risk—only to later discover a problem that was undetectable at the time. And embryo 2, which you passed over, would have avoided this outcome … had you only chosen differently.

Why does having more choice lead to more regret? It's because the brain chronically simulates possible futures. You can't help this; it happens under the hood, without your awareness. The brain doesn't live in real time: it constantly simulates from what-is to what-could-be. And it spends much of its time simulating what-could-have-been: the world that would have existed had you made different choices. Such fictive outcomes are compared against actual outcomes—and the difference is experienced as regret or relief. This is one way we learn. We use the signals of regret and relief to update our models of the world, and this helps us navigate our choices the next time a similar situation arises.

In the 1950s, psychologist Herbert Simon pointed out that many people act as "maximizers"—that is, we want to make sure we always make the best possible choice. Unfortunately, as the number of options increases, it becomes ever more difficult to know that we've made the optimal pick. It is theorized that much of modern anxiety comes from the increased opportunities for selection, at the cost of happiness.

When it comes to offspring, we have always had a simplicity born of choicelessness. Now, more and more couples will opt out of that. This is not to say we shouldn't build more choice into our lives; in this case, it will allow us to birth generations with less disease. But when things that were formerly out of our control become within our control, we'll have to be poised for a somewhat different emotional world: one with the peculiar juxtaposition of more healthy, beautiful children, and more parental remorse.

61

Following spread: Sculptures by Sun-Rae Kim, part of a series called *Tscho-Young Nina's Friends.*

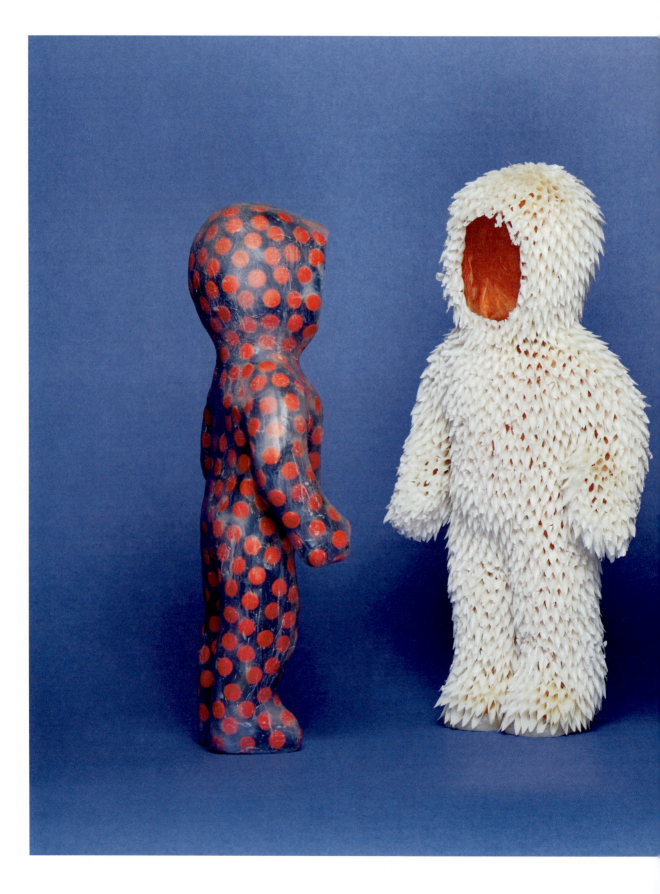

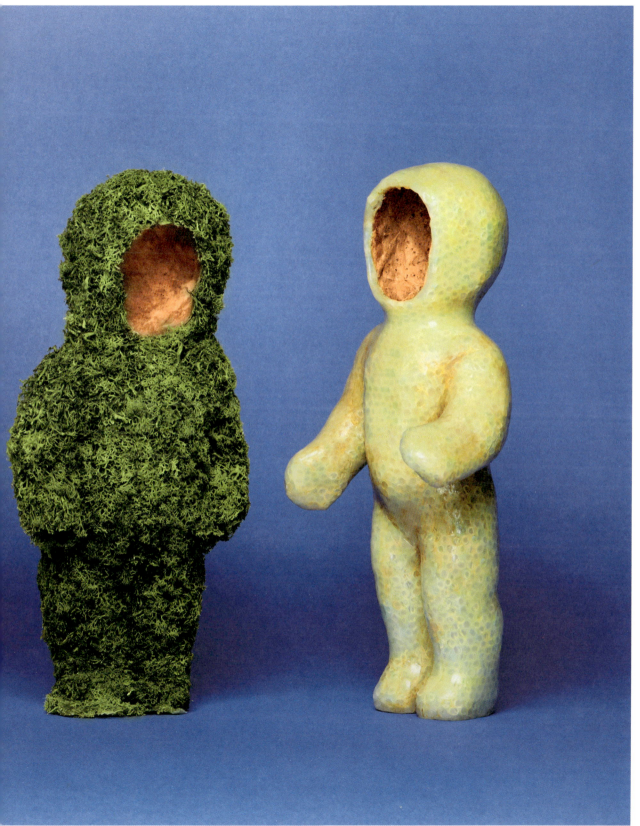

Zack Denfeld
Cathrine Kramer
Emma Conley
Unhinged, Bonkers, and Delicious

Unhinged, Bonkers, and Delicious

Zackery Denfeld, Cathrine Kramer, and Emma Conley are artists who collaborate with scientists, chefs, biohackers, and farmers to "prototype alternative culinary futures"—ideally ones in which food production is "more just, biodiverse, and beautiful."

We launched the Center for Genomic Gastronomy in 2010 to document the biotechnologies and biodiversity of human food systems from the perspective of the eater. It began as a bit of a satire of molecular gastronomy, which we felt was too focused on chemistry, modernity, and abstraction. We wanted to help eaters feel less alienated from the organisms and environments that are manipulated by our food cultures.

We present our research in the form of recipes, meals, publications, lectures, and exhibitions. We've put pop-up food carts on the streets of such cities as New York, Dublin, Panaji, and Edinburgh so we could quickly assemble organisms, ingredients, and human eaters in new configurations. For example, we rolled out a Smog Synthesizer, which simulates "aeroir," the smell and flavor of air pollution from various places and times. Our De-Extinction Deli is a fantastical market stand designed to highlight the emerging technologies, risks, and outcomes of the movement to revive, rear, and possibly eat extinct species. The Seed-O-Matic, the world's slowest vending machine, dispenses heirloom seeds and small bags of soil.

We use these carts to open up conversations about what values and attributes eaters want in their food and the systems that produce it. The carts are vehicles for dreaming about the future of food, prototyping it through taste, and activating culinary and ecological desires. It is especially important to make food that is both unexpected and delicious. Taste matters. Conviviality over food, taking pleasure in the daily rituals of eating, is one of the things that makes us human. Eating should connect us with each other and be pleasurable and joyous.

Let's talk about some food futures that we don't see as pleasurable and joyous.

Supplying mega cities with massive vats of lab-grown meat, automated vertical farms, and algae tanks does not seem beautiful, biodiverse, or delicious. Those visions abstract and standardize food and minimize seasonal variation and geographic particularities. On the other hand, imagining that everyone in the future will be supplied by glorified victory gardens and farmers markets is not much better. That dream is based on an idealized notion of how we actually grow and eat our food today. We need to imagine futures that

Shown right: This meringue cookie was made with smoggy air created in the Center for Genomic Gastronomy's Smog Synthesizer. The artists combined chemicals and exposed them to UV light to roughly recreate the smog in London in the 1800s and 1900s.

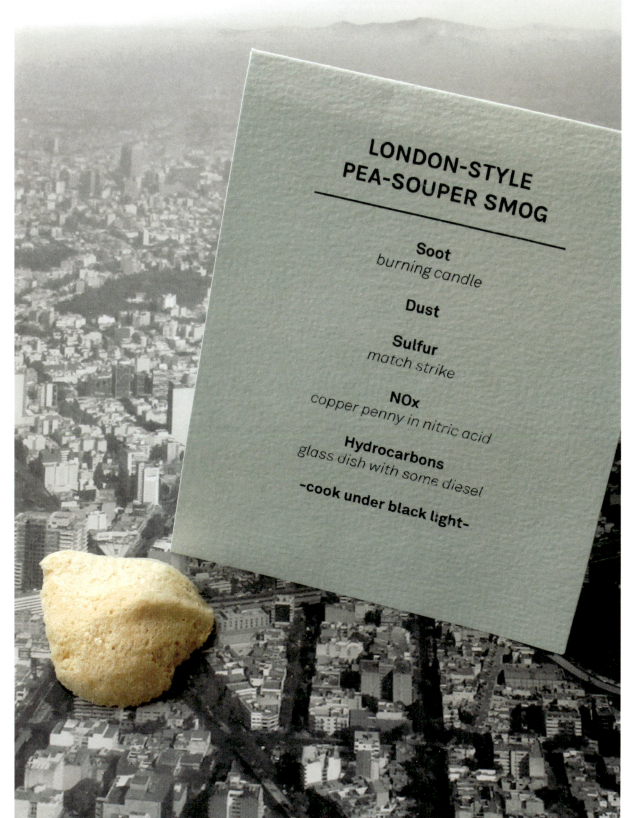

LONDON-STYLE
PEA-SOUPER SMOG

Soot
burning candle

Dust

Sulfur
match strike

NOx
copper penny in nitric acid

Hydrocarbons
glass dish with some diesel

-cook under black light-

Courtesy of the Center for Genomic Gastronomy

are more unhinged and bonkers than we have come to expect from sterile science fiction or foodie goody two shoes.

A good place to start is by eating some surprising ingredients, to see what they inspire. In these early days of the life science revolution, truth is stranger than fiction. By collaborating with scientists, chefs, biohackers, and farmers, we've used transgenic zebrafish in glowing sushi, air pollution in smog meringue tastings, and mutation-bred fruits in a BBQ sauce we called Cobalt-60 Sauce. When we serve ingredients like these to beta-tasters, they usually feel uncomfortable, start laughing, or both. That makes us happy, because laughter is a good indicator that people have been knocked off balance, are unable to rely on their conditioned expectations, and are thinking or seeing in a new way. Laughing induces open mouths and open minds. The Center for Genomic Gastronomy is happy to play the roles of mad scientist, mad chef, and trickster all at once.

We are now entering another phase of our work, looking at both very small and very large scales, across geographies. In our ArtMeatFlesh cooking show, we cook with the raw ingredients that are used for in-vitro meat. In pop-up Endophyte Clubs, we're isolating the microorganisms that live inside plants and creating recipes for an entirely new agro-ecosystem based on bio-pesticides. In our Planetary Sculpture Supper Club, we create dishes that document the ways planetary patterns change in response to how and what humans eat. Fad diets (like paleo) and culinary trends (such as the rise of nut-milks) can ripple through agricultural landscapes, changing how water and land are used in only a few years. If we are going to sculpt the entire planet with our eating habits, we might as well get good at it. Unfortunately, humans are doing pretty poorly with prevention and mitigation right now, so we are also investigating adaptation, preparing ingredients that have been impacted by increasingly frequent and severe wildfires.

Tools being developed in biology will let people reinvent food systems at every scale. But what values, preferences, and desires will drive this reinvention? It is unlikely that it will resemble the totalizing diagrams used when dreaming up the "cities of tomorrow." Instead, we envision fractal futures that look like a collection of recipe cards that can be tried, amended, and added to. Fractal futures are non-linear and messy and require connecting, tinkering, and feedback across many scales. From biology to art. From plant breeder to chef. From farm to plate to planet, and back again.

Shown right: A postcard used in the De-Extinction Deli, a market stand that prompts discussions about reviving vanished species. Visitors can write and mail pre-addressed postcards to leading researchers and thinkers in the field of de-extinction.

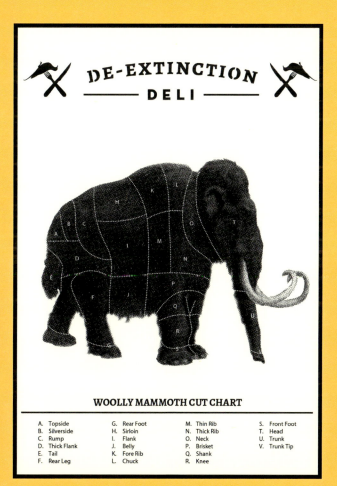

DE-EXTINCTION
— DELI —

WOOLLY MAMMOTH CUT CHART

A. Topside	G. Rear Foot	M. Thin Rib	S. Front Foot
B. Silverside	H. Sirloin	N. Thick Rib	T. Head
C. Rump	I. Flank	O. Neck	U. Trunk
D. Thick Flank	J. Belly	P. Brisket	V. Trunk Tip
E. Tail	K. Fore Rib	Q. Shank	
F. Rear Leg	L. Chuck	R. Knee	

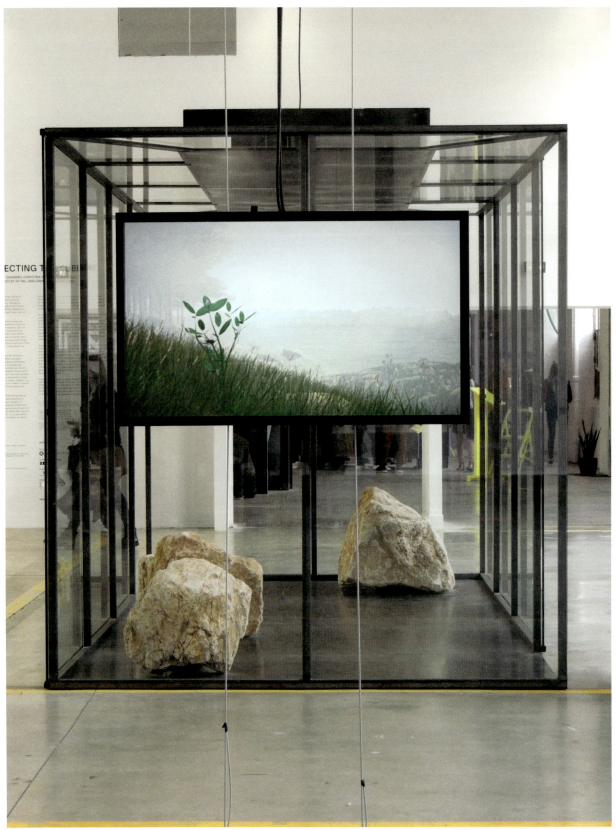

Christina Agapakis
Sissel Tolaas
Daisy Ginsberg
Resurrecting the Sublime

Resurrecting the Sublime

What would an extinct flower smell like? That question drove Christina Agapakis, a molecular biologist and artist, to take a list of 116 extinct plants to the Harvard Herbaria and look for preserved specimens. She ultimately found 14 of the plants on her list and persuaded the custodian to let her snip tiny samples off the ancient specimens. Engaging in a brilliant bit of what Stephan Schuster of Penn State University named "museomics," Agapakis shipped the samples off to the Paleogenomics Lab at UC Santa Cruz to extract their DNA.

The genes that encode the enzymes for floral scent molecules are generally about 1,700 letters long. But the longest strands of DNA the Santa Cruz scientists were able to extract were only about 50 letters. Luckily, the differences between the genomes of one plant and another are not so great. Using the genes of other plants as references, a computational biologist at Gingko Bioworks, the synthetic biology company where Agapakis is creative director, was able to fill in the blanks.

The next step was to embed the DNA assembled from the various plants in *Saccharomyces cerevisiae* (brewer's yeast) and coax it into expressing unique scent compounds. Sissel Tolaas, an olfactory artist based in Berlin, worked to balance the scents of those various molecules to generate a fragrance associated with each plant.

Conceptual artist Alexandra Daisy Ginsberg designed an immersive art installation using vitrines, smell diffusers, animation, and boulders to depict the landscape. Visitors can walk up and smell fragrances that otherwise might have been lost. It has been displayed at the Centre Pompidou in Paris and the Milan Triennial. The whole project is an elegant blend of art and science that inspires us to consider what we've lost, and whether and how we could recover it. Is resurrecting extinct species a utopian dream?

Agapakis says the project is a reminder that technology can be regenerative and not purely extractive. However, her collaborator Ginsberg wonders: "Why do we focus on creating new life forms and preserving and extending human life when we're so intricately tied up with other bits of the natural world and are unable to actually motivate ourselves to protect it?"

Previous spread: Installation view of *Resurrecting the Sublime* at the Biennale Internationale Design Saint-Étienne, 2019. *Orbexilum stipulatum* (vitrine with smell diffusion, limestone boulders, animation, ambient soundscape).

Shown right: *Orbexilum stipulatum,* also known as the Falls-of-the-Ohio Scurfpea, was an extinct legume last seen on Rock Island, near Louisville, Kentucky, in 1881. Its habitat was subsequently flooded by a dam built in the 1920s.

Following spread, left: Installation view of *Resurrecting the Sublime* at *Better Nature*, Vitra Design Museum Gallery, 2019. *Leucadendron grandiflorum* (Salisb.) R. Br. (smell diffusion hood, granite boulder, animation).

Following spread, right: Digital reconstruction of the *Leucadendron grandiflorum* (Salisb.) R. Br. on Wynberg Hill, behind Table Mountain, Cape Town, South Africa, prior to its last sighting in 1806.

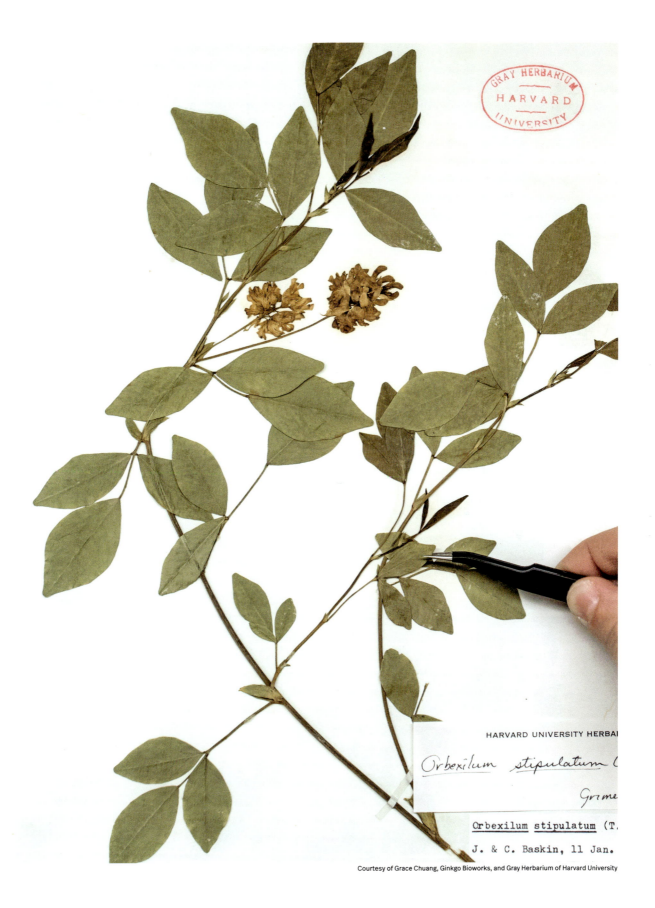

HARVARD UNIVERSITY HERBAR

Orbexilum stipulatum (

Grime

<u>Orbexilum</u> <u>stipulatum</u> (T.

J. & C. Baskin, 11 Jan.

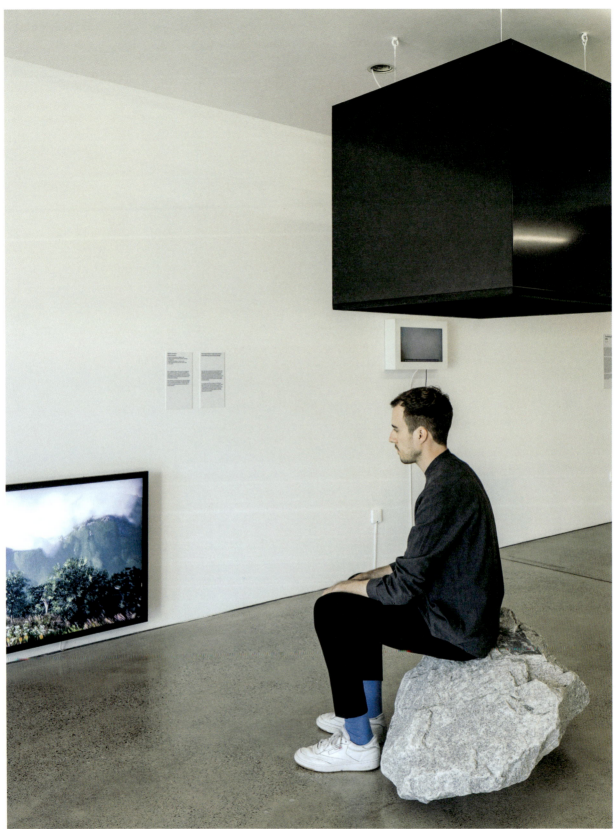

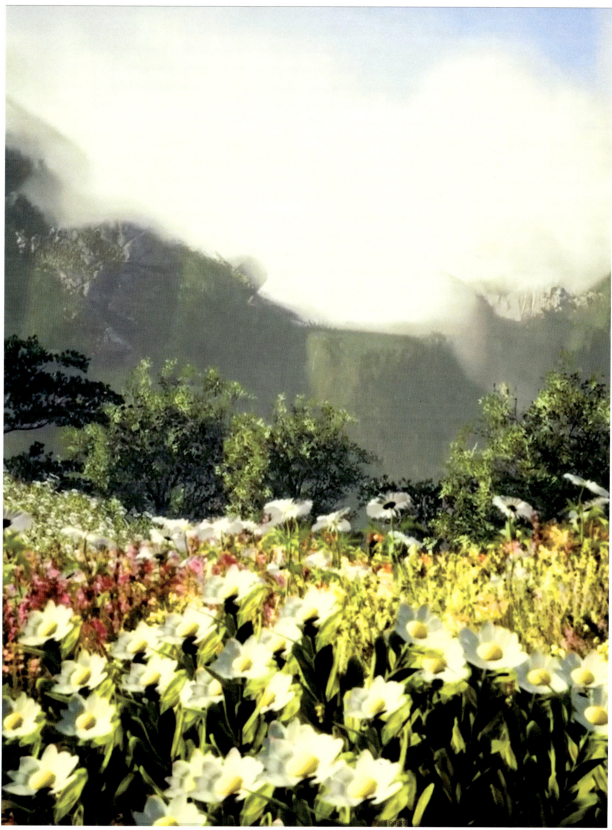

Samira Kiani

My CRISPR Safety Checklist

My CRISPR Safety Checklist

Samira Kiani is a geneticist and synthetic biologist who is opening a new lab at the University of Pittsburgh in 2020. She's also a producer of *The Human Game*, a documentary about gene editing.

I focus on developing tools that control the safety of CRISPR-based gene therapies. How can we actually engineer safety and controllability mechanisms into CRISPR?

We are working on a few different aspects. One of them is to modify the Cas9 protein so it doesn't provoke an immune response in the body. We're developing safety switches, so we will be able to control the activity of Cas9 in the tissues we want or at the times we want. We're even looking into applying CRISPR for epigenetic therapy rather than just creating permanent changes in DNA by gene editing. The theme of all of these is: How can we can make CRISPR safer so that it can be translated faster for clinical trials?

We have a moral responsibility not to deprive future generations of these technologies. But we need to be very creative in controlling the risks. Eventually, I'd like to see even more safety mechanisms. These are things that aren't technically possible yet, like the ability to track whatever DNA we change. That would be tricky, ethically, in human beings; you don't want to be able to mark people who are genetically modified and thus distinct from society. But it would be beneficial to understand which individual animals, like flies or mosquitoes, are genetically modified.

Or imagine the ability to reverse whatever we change in DNA. The ability to shut down or destroy one of our gene edits if an adverse reaction happens. Or the ability to limit its expression or activity to a time or location we want, whether it's inside the body or even a particular location in the world. Ideally, we would develop a capacity to dispatch countermeasure strategies such as safety kits to every household.

These are things we want to imagine for a technology like this that moves fast and spreads fast.

As told to Brian Bergstein

Shown right: Engineered human liver tissue derived from stem cells and enhanced by CRISPR.

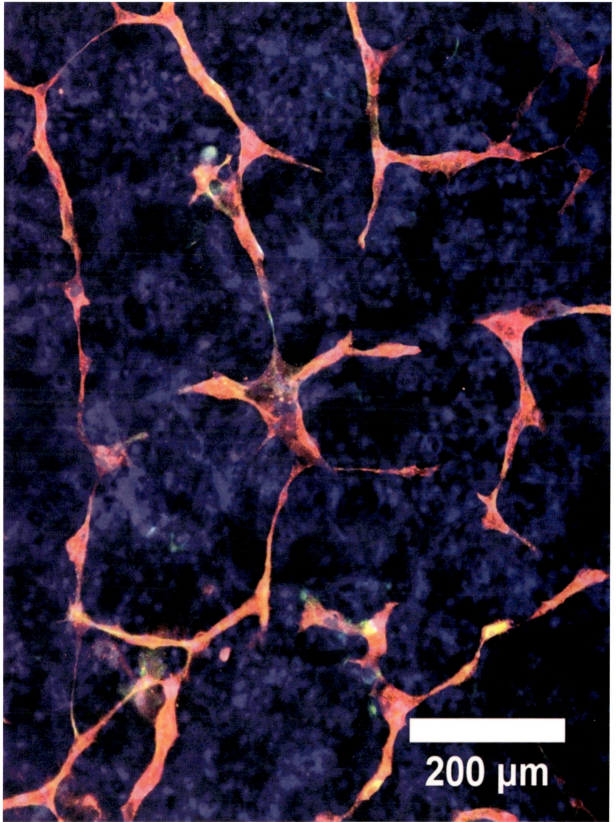

200 μm

"When we alter the fundamental building blocks that make up who we are, we are also changing the nature of our humanity. But we shouldn't fear it as being unnatural. We should think of it as a gift, a chance to design our legacy."
DAISY ROBINTON | MOLECULAR BIOLOGIST

Bowen Zhao

Your Custom-Made Microbiome

Your Custom-Made Microbiome

Bowen Zhao was 17 when he began working at BGI-Shenzhen, the world's largest genome-sequencing company. Before long he was leading a group that mined DNA data for the genetic roots of human intelligence. Today he is running a startup in Beijing called QuantiHealth, which hopes to develop personalized ways of fine-tuning your microbiome, which is the collection of microbes in your body and greatly affects your health and well-being. Journalist Yiting Sun interviewed Zhao for NEO.LIFE.

Why did you stop researching the genetics of intelligence?
The purpose of that project was to explore the boundaries of genome sequencing's application. The technology was getting cheaper and cheaper, so we wanted to know what it can bring for ordinary consumers. I didn't fully appreciate the weight of the project in the realm of ethics back then.

Human cognitive abilities are a highly complex matter, and to get to the bottom of their genetic basis, we needed to study genetic variants in at least 2,000 individuals with high IQ. The cost of gathering these samples exceeded the actual cost of sequencing. We decided not to devote more resources to this project, even though it didn't formally come to an end. There are many reasons for this decision. BGI is an enterprise, and this is not something an enterprise should be doing.

Why did you decide there was an opportunity in personalized health care?
Because for so long, genome sequencing focused on determining the nature of something: What species is it and what's the sequence of its DNA? My work at BGI obviously centered around this.

Let's say I've got a biological sample, and I feed it into a sequencing machine to digitize it. The data file I get contains lots of information, but where are the most valuable bits? Many people would assume that they are in the sequence, but that is more or less true only when studying one species. We've collected so many human saliva samples, but we've paid the most attention to the human genome in these samples, and have completely failed to consider the other things in these samples.

How can you change health care by cataloging the DNA in our microbiomes?
Three applications come to mind.

One is the diagnosis and prediction of many chronic metabolic disorders. The second is pinpointing the cause of infections. In many cases, today's doctors can't find the specific microbes that are causing infections, and even if they can, the result only becomes available after several days. By then the doctor would have already prescribed an antibiotic based on an educated guess in order to save the patient's life. And if one kind doesn't work, the doctor would switch to another one. This kind of abuse of antibiotics increases the likelihood that microbes will become resistant. I believe we could find the exact pathogen within 24 hours by quantifying the microbial DNA in samples from patients.

The third application is creating a new class of pharmaceuticals based on the chemicals produced by microbes' metabolic processes.

But there will be other applications that I haven't thought of yet.

Probiotic pills and drinks apparently don't work very well. Do you expect to come up with more targeted probiotic products?
What's really influencing your health is the entire microbiome, not specific kinds of bacteria. If I only have one type of probiotic in my body, and all the other bacteria have died, I'd be really sick.

To address this issue, first you need to figure out the interactions between the microbiome and the human body. This is what we are trying to do with the reference database we are putting together. We want to identify and culture as many kinds of microbes that live in and on the human body as possible. And then we want to discover their functions.

Many doctors are administering fecal microbiota transplants (FMT), but to my mind, this is akin to transfusing blood before even knowing what blood types are. Once we have the reference database, we don't need to do fecal microbiota transplants anymore. We could do "artificial microbiome transplants." When we have enough types of living bacteria that make up the human microbiome in our reference database, we could personalize the proportions of bacteria. That means we could synthesize the microbiome of anyone in the world, even a microbiome that doesn't exist yet. This is the 2.0 version of today's FMT.

"Every hacker I know does a ton of outreach, but really,
governments should fund community labs and encourage
citizens to participate as a civic duty."
MEOW-LUDO DISCO GAMMA MEOW-MEOW | BIOHACKER

Robert Plomin

Shake Up Education Using DNA

Shake Up Education Using DNA

Robert Plomin, a professor in the Institute of Psychiatry, Psychology, and Neuroscience at King's College London, is renowned for his decades of research on twins and adopted children, which examined how heredity and environment shape human behavior. His most recent book is *Blueprint: How DNA Makes Us Who We Are*.

Inherited differences in DNA are becoming more and more powerful predictors of physical and physiological traits. This essential insight, which I call the DNA revolution, is sweeping through medicine, making it possible for health care to move toward prevention rather than cure. That is, rather than waiting until someone gets a heart attack, it is surely better in every way—medically, economically, personally—to prevent heart attacks.

The same logic holds as well for psychology, my area of research. In just the last three years, DNA has also begun to serve as a predictor of traits like depression, schizophrenia, and school achievement, and the effects of the DNA revolution will soon be seen here too.

Prevention requires prediction, and DNA is a unique predictor. We begin life as a single cell with half of our DNA from our mother and half from our father. All of our trillions of cells have a set of DNA codes that is almost identical to the ones in that primordial cell. So, DNA can predict heart attacks just as well from conception or birth as it can predict in later life.

This is why the U.K. Health Secretary, Matt Hancock, has put the DNA revolution at the top of his agenda for transforming the National Health Service. It's said that a severe heart attack costs the NHS £700,000, not to mention the suffering and lost quality of life. Preventing problems rather than waiting until the problems emerge could be the economic salvation of the NHS. (In contrast, I don't see how insurance-based health systems as in the U.S. can survive the DNA revolution. If you have a high genetic risk for heart attacks, you would be asked to pay a higher premium, just as automobile insurance costs more for individuals at higher risk, such as young males and people who have had accidents.)

If we're going to use DNA to predict and prevent medical problems, we could do the same in education. Surely it is better to protect a child from developing reading problems than waiting until the child goes to school and fails to learn to read. Reading problems cause a lot of collateral damage to children's attitudes toward school and toward themselves.

It's hard to put Humpty Dumpty back together once he's fallen off the wall.

Most children who have reading problems in school had language problems in early child-hood. There are good interventions for language problems, but in general, you get what you pay for. More intensive, and thus more expensive, interventions have a better chance of success. But we cannot afford expensive preventive interventions for everyone. If we can target individuals at high genetic risk, it would be cost effective to provide them extended one-on-one help.

Similarly, it must be better to predict and mitigate behavioral problems such as atten-tional and hyperactivity problems, which occupy as much of teachers' time and energy and cause as much angst as learning problems. Attempts to lessen these problems on the cheap–using the internet, for example–have at best small and temporary effects.

Such targeted use of the most expensive interventions is becoming possible because of what we call polygenic scores. A century of research on twins and children who were adopted has built a mountain of evidence showing that inherited DNA differences con-tribute importantly to our individuality–our personality, mental health, and cognition. Traits such as cognitive abilities (e.g., verbal ability and memory), school-related skills (reading and mathematics), and behavioral problems (attention and activity level) are as heritable as common medical problems (high blood pressure, type 2 diabetes). What's new is that we are now able to use polygenic scores to predict such variations in behavior by analyzing thousands of DNA differences associated with a trait.

For example, my team has shown that we can now predict 15% of the variance between children in their scores on the GCSE, a test administered to U.K. children at the end of compulsory schooling at age 16. Fifteen percent may sound small overall, but this is a stronger predictor than parental income. (The strongest predictor is the child's own educational attainment before the test, but that's not knowable at birth.) And the predic-tive power of this polygenic score can be seen most clearly at the extremes. For example, 75% of children in the top 10% of DNA scores for educational achievement go on to university, whereas only 25% of children in the lowest 10% go to university.

When I wrote my book *Blueprint: How DNA Makes Us Who We Are*, I hoped that the zeitgeist had shifted away from environmentalism–which is the view that we are what we learn–to a more balanced view that recognizes the importance of nature. And I was relieved by the overall positive reaction to the book. However, some criticisms emerged. The most common one is that the book leads to fatalism, the notion that if our genes are so important, we have to accept our fates. To critics, the word "blueprint" in the book's title and my light-hearted description of DNA as a "fortune teller" connote determinism. But genes are not destiny for common disorders like heart attacks nor for complex traits like school performance.

Genes are hard-wired and deterministic for single-gene disorders such as Huntington disease, which causes neural degeneration and early death. That is, the genetic variant for Huntington disease is necessary and sufficient—if you have that variant you will die from the disease unless something else kills you first. But for more common disorders and complex traits, the genetic influence comes from thousands of tiny DNA effects. These are probabilistic propensities rather than predetermined programs.

In *Blueprint* I wrote that "Parents matter but they don't make a difference," which was often misconstrued. In the populations studied so far, with their mix of genetic and environmental differences, variations in inherited DNA emerge as the major systematic force in shaping who we are as individuals. These variations are more important than differences in parenting. But to say that parents do not make a difference in children's outcomes on average, in a particular population at a particular time, does not mean that parents *cannot* make a difference. DNA does not predict all that could be or prescribe what should be.

Like other major advances in science, the DNA revolution has potential for harm as well as for good. There are many issues that need to be discussed, such as the responsible use of these polygenic DNA scores. But I am a cheerleader for using them because I see many benefits of being able to predict problems and promise from early in life.

Shown right: Various readouts of electrical activity in the brain, recorded by EEG.

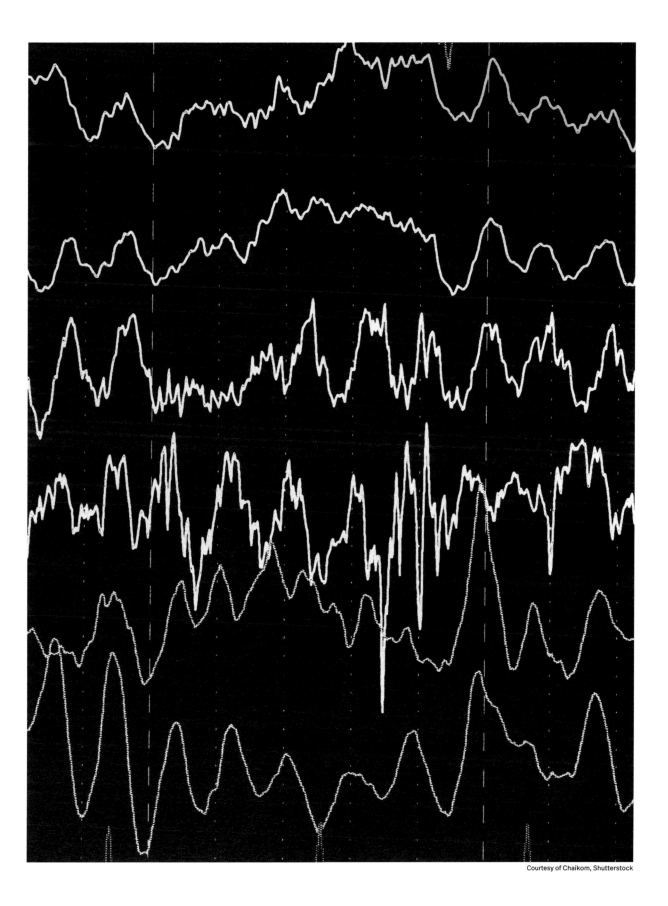

Changle Zhou

Brain-Machine Interfaces Will Boost Brains and Machines

Brain-Machine Interfaces Will Boost Brains and Machines

Changle Zhou is a professor in the Department of Artificial Intelligence at Xiamen University in Fujian, China. In one of his research projects, human volunteers wear EEG caps while they watch videos of humanoid robots dancing or performing other actions. Zhou hopes this lays the groundwork for systems in which people control machines with their thoughts.

For the past 30 years or so, I've been trying to infuse human-like intelligence into machines. But even after I designed AI algorithms that can understand metaphors and compose music—intellectual pursuits unique to humans—I still felt that something was missing in these seemingly intelligent machines.

Sure, these machines are capable of crunching lots of data in a short amount of time. But their computational prowess is also their Achilles heel: Try giving them a task that lacks any rules or logical explanations, and they immediately malfunction. A computer is not capable of describing the emotion it experiences upon hearing its own music composition, because it doesn't experience any. Qualia, which are humans' internal experiences aroused by sensory inputs, defy logic. And it's this quality of human intelligence that I hold dearest.

Brain-machine interfaces can bridge this gap between human and machine intelligence by creating a kind of "mixed intelligence." The human component in this mixed intelligence doesn't have to be a real person—it could be living neurons sustained outside human bodies. After building two-way communication between these neurons and a computer, we then have a system that can both handle massive amounts of computation and have subjective experiences. This system is not a human, but it's not just a passive machine, either.

Mixed intelligence will improve our lives in ways that were unimaginable before. Try to picture the joy on a paralyzed person's face when that person can send a robot with mixed intelligence to go to a party! Through wireless communication with a robot, a housebound person can see new faces, hear new stories, and most importantly, rediscover the excitement of socializing. By the same token, if robots can understand love and other kinds of wonderful emotions humans experience, they'll become better caregivers. I believe all the intelligent systems we develop should serve humanity, and this kind of mixed intelligence is no exception.

We could engineer the neurons in different ways to suit our various needs, which means we don't need to incorporate all the different kinds of subjective experiences a human can experience into one system. We could design one type of mixed intelligence that is capable of stirring up emotions in itself, and yet another type that has a sense of its own existence and knows that it's different from other systems.

The potential for this powerful technology to be used for evil purposes is huge. I don't want to see cases where it's used to control you or alter your temperament. So how do we ensure that mixed intelligence will become a force that helps us prosper? My answer is the right education and nurturing—not just for people, but for machines with mixed intelligence, too.

Many education systems put too much emphasis on measuring and enhancing intelligence, but fail to reward other qualities that foster humanity's collective well-being. It's time to fix this. When the heart is benevolent—be it the human heart or the heart of mixed intelligence—society will be good, and people will stay away from evil deeds.

As told to Yiting Sun

Siranush Babakhanova

Students for a Better Life

Students for a Better Life

Siranush Babakhanova is an MIT undergraduate, class of 2020, who is majoring in physics and computer science. She also is a researcher in the Synthetic Neurobiology Group.

I've spent many sleepless nights in simultaneous grief and excitement about the current direction and potential future of human beings. I keep thinking about technologies for human enhancement that are available now or will soon emerge—technologies that are likely to have great or severe implications.

I craved a community where I could learn from experts in relevant disciplines, discuss solutions, and induce actions. Luckily, I happened to meet a number of inquisitive and forward-thinking individuals at MIT who convinced me to form this cross-disciplinary community. My cofounder Logan Ford and I call the group Xapiens: sapiens for wise being and "X" for the unknown.

From transportation to modern medicine, from gadgets to weapons, all the technologies humans have made to explore the world and make their lives better (or worse) are, in fact, enhancements. Whether they allow us to fly, get immunity against pathogens, communicate with each other over long distances, or kill each other in big numbers, all technologies allow us to transcend limitations that were previously inherent in being human. But present-day Earthlings are at a critical turning point because of new biotechnologies, non-biological intelligences, and the exploration of space and other extreme environments. We're now developing technologies that will allow more drastic changes than ever in the way we live. We at Xapiens feel a responsibility to steer these human enhancements in ways that mitigate existential, ecological, and societal risks, not only for us but for our kin on this planet. We seek ways to use these technologies to make our future better.

In particular, powerful biotechnological tools available today, such as gene editing, and ones that could come soon, like neural interfaces, might provide the most benefits to people with social and economic power, increasing the disparities between certain groups. This may cause a potentially non-rectifiable segregation of society, and entire populations may be left behind in the evolutionary race. Xapiens is looking for opportunities to use these technologies to decrease disparities instead.

We also believe that current developments in computer science suggest that there will be artificial general intelligence (AGI), and some future forms might outperform humans and be harmful to our species. If we are not ready by that time to evolve our biological hardware at a comparable pace or "merge" with cyber-intelligence, we may not have another chance to survive. Therefore, we are particularly interested in seeking new bio-cyber interfaces.

Finally, as humans begin exploring alternative environments in space and undergoing enhancements that make it possible to survive far from Earth, we want to monitor and influence the committees making decisions on who will be modified and how.

So far we have been mainly discussing the future of *Homo sapiens*. But we also are considering the Transhumanist Declaration from 1998. It advocates for the welfare of all sentience, including *in silico* intelligence, animals, and generations that will exist in the future. Xapiens also stands for the preservation of the archives and documents remaining from the lives of those who came before us, and the rights of any entities that decide to unite their intelligences, if a technology for a hive mind or something similar arises.

Finally, human enhancement is about more than just survival. It expands us and lets us experience new forms of beauty, joy, love, and compassion. In hopes of saturating our lives with these experiences, people write music, paint, and engage in mathematics. We sleep and see beautiful and beautifully terrifying dreams, and the beauty in the organization of the universe allows us to hypothesize about its laws. We often imagine no end to the amount of beauty and love that exists. Enhancing ourselves may well allow us to experience this at its fullest—in all the senses, at all scales, and dimensions.

97

Through enhancement, humans can transcend new cosmic, mental, and societal horizons. I would like to hear the heartbeat of the stars and resonate with the fluctuating fabric of space-time as if it were the lining of my own body. I can envision a convoluted cosmic dance and memories of civilizations of creatures and their love and hate stories embedded in my subconsciousness. It would involve some poetic intrigue or tragedy, because I find that beautiful too. I want to experience all that, and I see Xapiens as a way to get there. Instead of trying to predict the future, I choose to participate in architecting it to be as beautiful as it can be.

Acknowledgments: Xapiens is funded by the MIT Division of Student Life, the MIT Media Lab, and the McGovern Institute for Brain Research. I thank Alexi Choueiri, Loyd Hoyt Waites, Nathan Rollins, Afika Nyati, and Brody West for their feedback on these ideas.

Kristen Fortney

Longevity Is Just Getting Started

Longevity Is Just Getting Started

Kristen Fortney is founder and CEO of BioAge, which is pinpointing biological mechanisms of aging that might be addressable with new drugs. Using human blood samples that have been stored in "biobanks" for decades, the company is analyzing how proteins, metabolites, and other molecular signals differ in the samples taken from people who went on to live the longest, healthiest lives.

I'm pretty confident that molecules that I've already seen under development are going to add something like 10 to 20 years to the human lifespan. And that's a conservative lower bound on what we can see in the future. There's no obvious limit in physics or biology on how long a person can live. There are examples of mammals, like bowhead whales, that can live longer than humans can. Those whales live into their 200s.

There have been major increases in average life expectancy over the last century, but they have come from things like clean water, antibiotics, and lowered infant mortality. The maximum lifespan hasn't really moved much at all. Discoveries that we can actually delay aging are all quite new. The first time that an intervention was shown to reproducibly make mice live longer, which means that lots of different labs did it, in hundreds of animals, was the drug rapamycin in 2009. That's brand new—the first drugs based on that discovery in mice are in human clinical trials now. They could be plausibly on the market in a few years.

That's just the first of these mechanisms that we really believe will move the needle on aging. There are going to be a lot more, because there are dozens of things that you can do to other species to make them live longer, and that should translate to us. Ideally we'll get to the point where someone is taking drugs when they're still healthy that will delay the onset of multiple diseases, the way that some people take statins today, or baby aspirins. It probably won't be all in one pill. There might be one pill targeting your aging immune system, another one targeting aging muscles. Some combination will be required to get some of those benefits.

Are there any potential downsides? You know, there's an old joke that science advances one funeral at a time as the old professors die off and are replaced. You can imagine power structures lasting longer, right? The thing is, though, this isn't going to happen overnight. I think it would be an issue if tomorrow we were all living to 1,000. That would be a really hard adjustment. But I don't think it's going to happen that way.

As told to Brian Bergstein

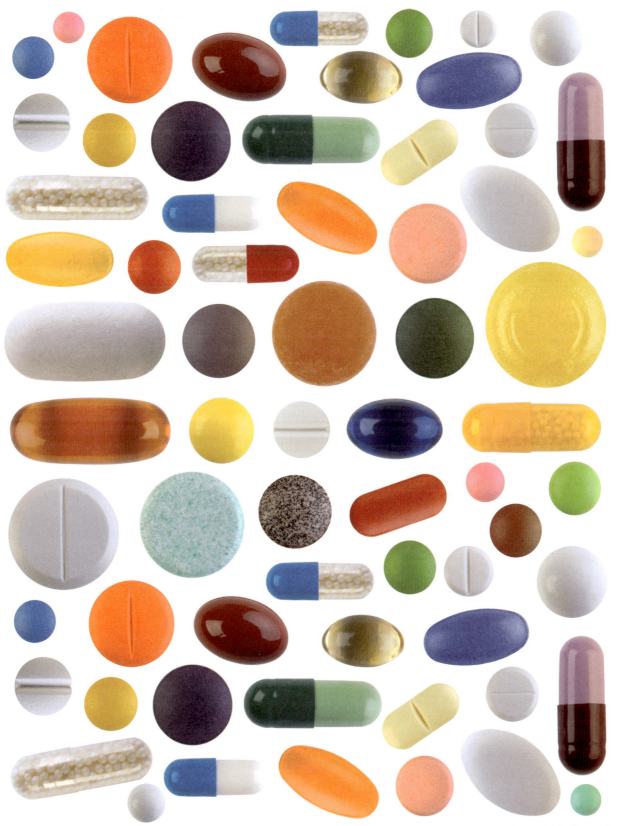

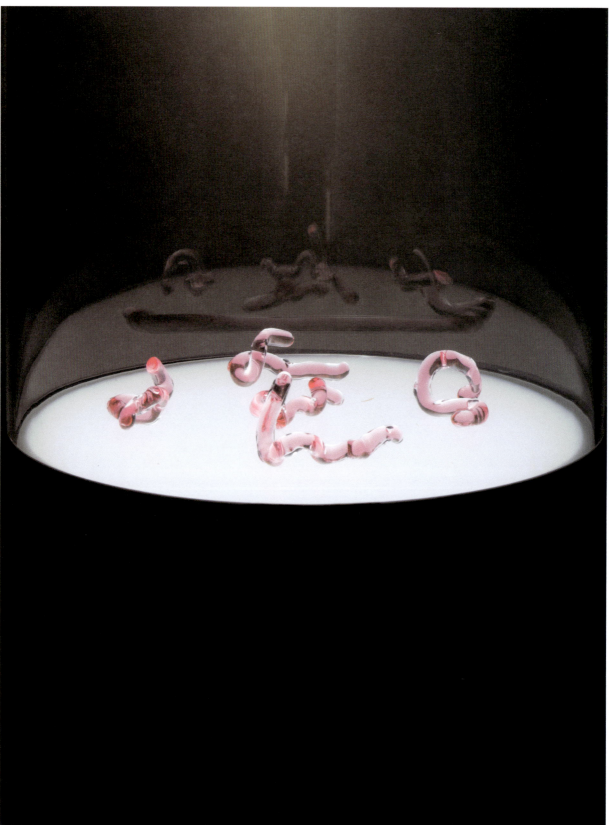

Heather
Dewey-Hagborg

Lovesick
Stranger Visions

Lovesick

Heather Dewey-Hagborg is an artist and biohacker in Brooklyn. In her work *Lovesick: The Transfection* (page 102), she imagines harnessing biotech to "spread affection and attachment and to combat the alienation and hate of the present." She collaborated with Integral Molecular, an antibody discovery company, to create a custom retrovirus designed to increase the production of oxytocin, a hormone that acts as a neurotransmitter in the brain. Oxytocin release is triggered by touch (such as hugging and breast feeding and orgasm) as well as social bonding, and has been shown to strengthen social memory in the brain.

The virus is contained in small glass vials the artist designed. The work is displayed alongside a video in which she and her partner sing a 14th century ballad about lovesickness. In place of the original Italian words, they sing the amino acid letters that correspond to the proteins in oxytocin. Singing the song and breaking the vial are intended to create a ritual worthy of the emotional upheaval to come. The virus, like a declaration of love or swallowing a cyanide pill, is meant to be irreversible.

Stranger Visions

In spite of her optimism about what we can do now and in the future, Dewey-Hagborg warns that we should not let ourselves be "tracked, analyzed, or cloned." To make her point, the artist extracted DNA from hair, cigarette butts, and discarded chewing gum she collected from streets and subways and public restrooms. Using forensic phenotyping techniques and extensive artistic license, she created life-sized, 3D-printed portrait masks of the unseen people who had left those things behind, prompting viewers to question the accuracy and ethics of this increasingly common police practice. In fact, the seven portraits in her show *Stranger Visions* (on the following pages) make these fictional people look like possible perpetrators in a police lineup.

Previous spread: *Lovesick* (2019); custom retrovirus, glass, two-channel video, music arranged by the artist. Installation view of *At the Temperature of My Body*, 2019.

Shown right and following spread: *Stranger Visions*, 2012-2013; Found genetic materials, custom software, 3D prints, documentation. Portrait dimensions: 8x6x6 inches.

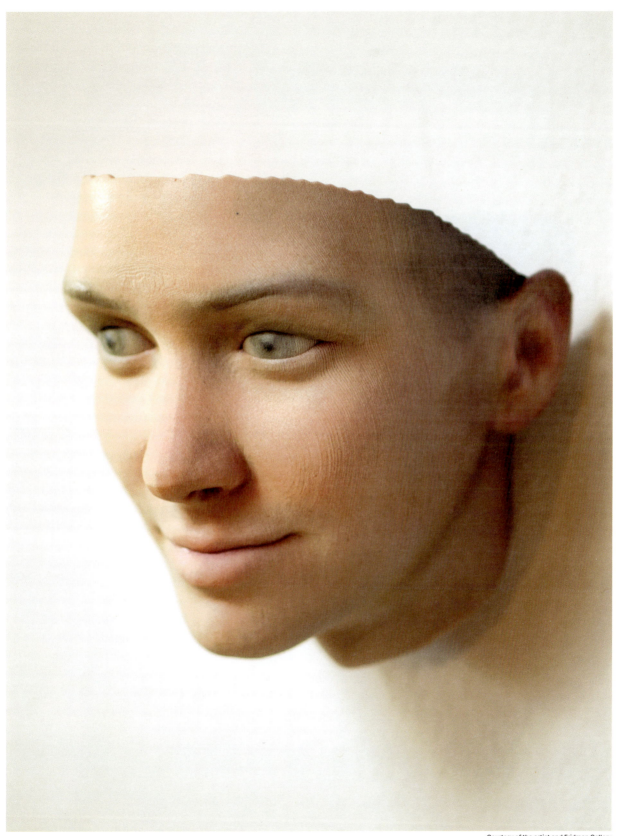

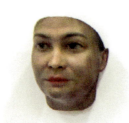
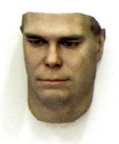
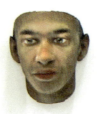

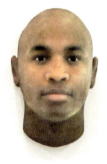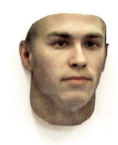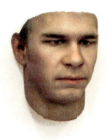

Megan Palmer

What Happens When Anyone Can Be a Bioengineer

What Happens When Anyone Can Be a Bioengineer

Megan Palmer, senior research scholar at the Center for International Security and Cooperation at Stanford, investigates strategies for managing the risks of emerging technologies. She founded the Synthetic Biology Leadership Excellence Accelerator Program (LEAP), and has devised social responsibility programs for the International Genetically Engineered Machine competition, known as iGEM.

In high school, my friends and I built a robot.

I was 16 and my fellow nerds and I convinced our physics teacher to help us register a team in Canada's chapter of the robotics competition known as FIRST. The rules were simple. Each team received a kit of parts and had to build a robot that fit inside a garbage can. Naturally, since this was Canada, it also had to play hockey. The grand prize went to the team whose hockey-playing robot won the most matches.

We convinced our parents' companies to sponsor our team while we scrambled to find designs that would enable our robot to hit a puck. The match was in Hamilton, Ontario, and we met kids from all over the country who shared our nerdy aspirations and our technical frustrations. It was fun and exciting, even though we placed nearly last. That wasn't surprising: I recall one teammate was more focused on getting our robot to spit fire than to hit a puck. Even without fire, we scared the judges by powering our bot with a pneumatic system. If too much pressure builds up, you have created an air-powered bomb.

Today, 16-year-olds can have a similar experience, but it isn't limited to robotics. Now they can build living machines. And I spend a lot of my time trying to ensure they aren't inspired to make the equivalent of a fire-spitting or air-bomb robot.

For the last 15 years, teams have participated in the International Genetically Engineered Machine (iGEM) competition, which was inspired by FIRST. The kits they get have DNA-encoded parts called biobricks. Instead of a garbage can, they have a choice of organisms (often *E. coli* or yeast, but other creatures, too) to serve as a "chassis." And in place of playing a game to win (which is a bad idea ... design your own pathogen!), they design a living machine to do something *useful*.

To win medals, iGEM teams must achieve goals such as creating new genetic components to add to the parts kit for subsequent years. They also compete for the best project—which could be anything from biomanufacturing a degradable plastic to engineering a biosensor for an environmental contaminant to prototyping a cell therapy. Every year thousands of people in hundreds of teams from dozens of countries descend on Boston for the competition. Their judges—volunteers from universities, companies, governments, and civil society—come to witness the future of biological engineering. My MIT classmates who competed in the first iGEM founded a company that's now worth more than $1 billion. They are designing custom organisms for everything from agriculture to cancer therapeutics.

But as tools and knowledge become more widely disseminated, I keep wondering what happens when any 16-year-old can engineer life. More than one bioengineer has mused, half-jokingly, that there will be dragons. But a dragon seems tame when you could build a pathogenic organism that could spread out of control. Disasters don't have to start with evil intent. I am just as concerned about an overeager do-gooder stumbling into dangerous territory.

Biology is not robotics. The stakes are higher and the principles are different: Biology reproduces, evolves, and directly interacts with other living things. But as in robotics, we discover and learn what is possible and permissible in part by playing around. So as we try to inspire the next generation of bioengineers, we also need to inspire them to be responsible. In iGEM, my fellow volunteers and I ask ourselves: *How can we encourage them to work on problems that matter? How can we enable the most important and exciting work to be done safely? How can we make it cooler to build a fire-fighting robot than a fire-spitting one?*

Our approach has been to codify these ethics in the competition's system of requirements and rewards. We call this the "human practices" part of the competition. Teams are incentivized to work with stakeholders on safety and other ethical issues coupled to their projects. These issues are complex; there is rarely a simple "best" approach. Responsible engineering is treated as a design challenge, and an essential component of any good project.

It is reassuring to watch teams embrace this challenge. Teams have worked with law enforcement to test the effectiveness of regulations that are meant to prevent people from purchasing dangerous DNA sequences. They have designed ways to control and trace the spread of their organisms. Teams have also engaged in policy forums in their home countries and at the United Nations. Dragons may intrigue them, but most people are equally interested in exploring how to make the world a better place.

Yet despite our best efforts to be proactive, there are always cases that cause alarm.

Sometimes teams use genetic components that are innocuous on their own but danger-ous when combined—like a part for delivery into a cell and a part that causes a cell to expand and burst (kind of like an air bomb!). This combination may be useful for finding and killing a cancer cell, but you don't want it going after healthy cells. Teams have also sought to test applications in animals, target pests, and design products that could cross national borders. Their projects often touch upon issues with limited or unequal precedent that have barely been considered by their senior mentors or governments.

As new issues arise, iGEM has made yearly revisions to the competition rules and evalu-ation system. Because working with young adults can appear to have lower stakes, iGEM has become a collaborative space for learning about how to govern bioengineering. In this setting, what often takes decades to enact in government policy can be tested on much faster time scales.

This doesn't mean that rules are never broken. As the competition has become bigger and projects have become more sophisticated, the rules have also needed enforcement. We now have dedicated "safety and security" and "responsible conduct" programs. We screen projects in advance to help the teams make adjustments, but these programs can also disqualify teams, as a few groups have learned the hard way. One time a team started a fire.

Which brings us back to the question: What happens when any 16-year-old can engineer life? People will always want to push boundaries, and when the wind blows the wrong way, even a small fire can lead to disaster.

To avoid a future spent constantly putting out fires, we must grow communities commit-ted to proactive and collaborative engagement with difficult issues. Our experience in the evolving experiment of "human practices" has taught us the power of positive incentives and elevating examples of good behavior. But it has also taught us that while self-gov-ernance is necessary, it is never going to be sufficient. We need to work with others to develop standards and ways to enforce them.

The world isn't a student competition. When kids grow up, they no longer respond to the T-shirts, stickers, and trophies that mean so much in iGEM. Biology can be lucrative as a platform for making almost anything. And the ability to manipulate biology is a powerful political force from the individual to the global scale. As we move toward a future when bioengineering can be practiced by anyone, we need to keep developing the culture and the incentives to ensure it is done for everyone.

Shown right: An artist's rendering of E. coli.

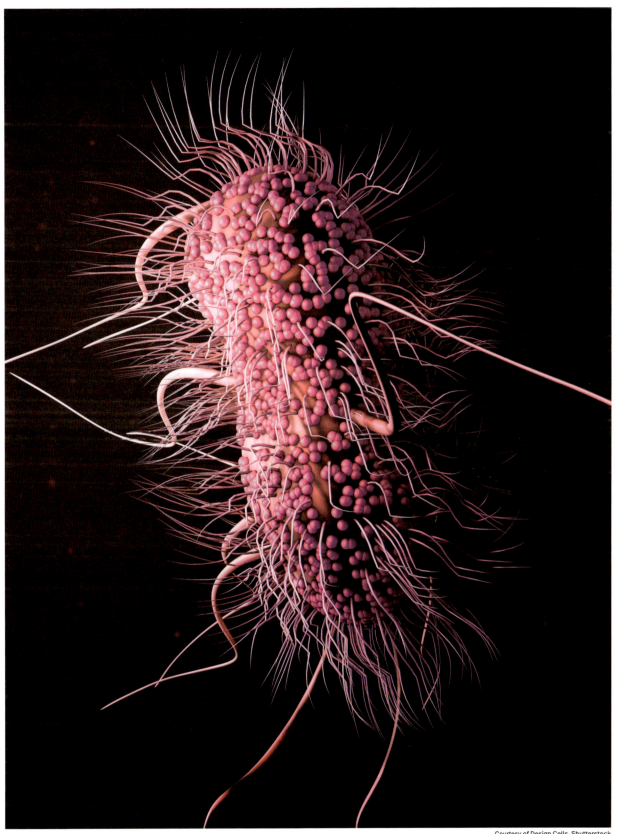

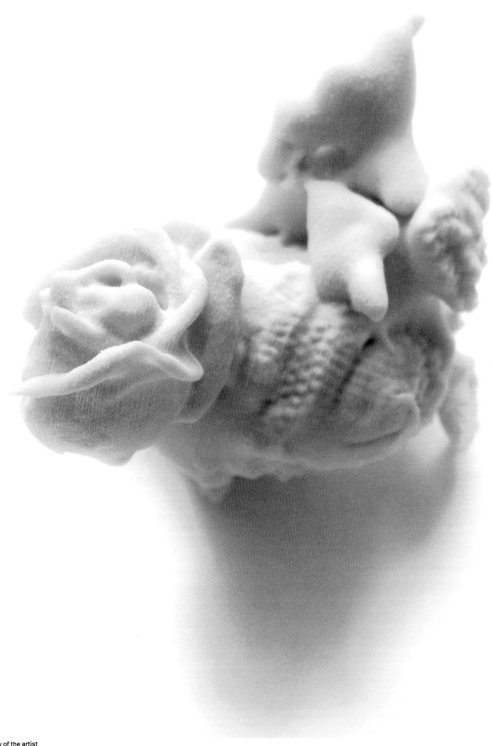

Becky Lyon
Fieldnotes from a Technobiocology

Fieldnotes from a Technobiocology

Becky Lyon is an artist in London who recently finished graduate studies at Central Saint Martins. She is the leader of an art research club, Elastic Nature, which explores what she describes as "the changing shape of nature."

If evolution is an exercise in recombining and reconfiguring existing material, does everything have the capacity to become a building block for life? Perhaps all matter, even that perceived as "synthetic," "expired," "dead," or "disposed," can be lively, expressive, and at some stage awakened. This is what I emphasize in a series of sculptures called *Fieldnotes from a Technobiocology*. What kinds of beings might emerge from the debris of DNA editing experiments? At the meeting point of nourishing earth and electrical waste? Where digital code meets biologic hardware?

Biopunks (page 114), made from 3D-printed plaster, are hybrid creatures that blend DNA from different species, potentially a combination of "natural" and "artificial" or gene-edited life forms. They display both recognizable features and alien traits. Were they designed this way in a lab? Or have wild and gene-edited organisms procreated? Are they wondrous expressions of human creativity or mutant monstrosities?

Skinterfaces and Sites of Material Exchange (opposite) is made of bioplastic on mesh. Here skin is a site of new kinds of activity. Biology and technology interface at the surface and materials metabolize; things grow, colors shape-shift. These transformations represent the exchanges that occur in the making, survival, and evolution of life. The work also questions to what extent living organisms are contained by their bodies and how extensively they are coupled with their surrounding medium.

In this new kind of "natural," I imagine phenomena such as bacteria ingesting and generating electricity from human pollution; photosynthesizing membranes sequestering carbon from the atmosphere; and new organisms using plastic as structural material. It all gestures toward a post-Anthropocene planet, with independent and self-generating systems free from human intervention. This presents a positive future trajectory in which the convergence of technology and biology results not in an abomination but an allegiance that helps to remediate and restore the planet.

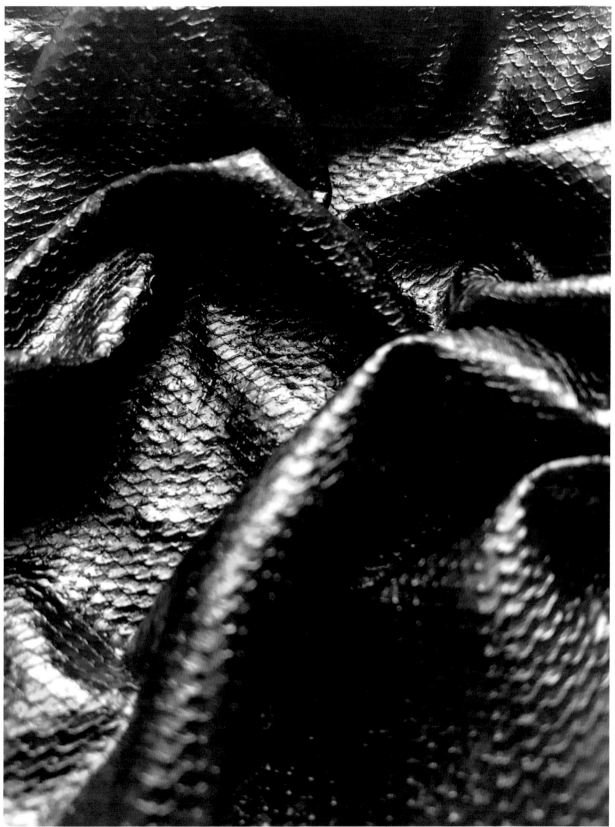

"I do not believe that tech should empathize with me. I don't want robots trying to emulate human qualities in any way. I'm looking for ways that technology enhances human capacity, and that's very different."

POPPY CRUM | NEUROSCIENTIST

Zoe Cormier

The Ideal Drug

The Ideal Drug

Zoe Cormier is a science journalist and the author of *Sex, Drugs & Rock 'n' Roll: The Science of Hedonism and the Hedonism of Science.*

There are hardly any cultures on the face of the Earth that have not indulged in narcotic pleasures. So universal is the behavior that UCLA psychopharmacologist Ronald Siegel once labeled our desire for intoxication the "fourth drive"—the first three being thirst, hunger, and sex.

Though most drugs can broadly be split into three categories—ones that get you stoned, stimulated, or tripped out—there are in fact countless reasons people do drugs: to stay awake, fall asleep, kill pain, deepen pleasure, inspire insights, dissolve egos, bond with others, delve inwards, provide clarity, explore consciousness, induce calm, spark excitement, prolong sex, return to innocence, expand visions, facilitate music, increase appetite, repress hunger, incite giggles, invoke tears. And in the future, people will do drugs for purposes we have not thought of yet.

Since humans became self-aware, we have used every available ingredient and technology in the pursuit of altered states. From the wild, leaves, flowers, roots, fungi, and even toad and scorpion venom have all been sampled. In the lab, gases, liquids, metals, and composites have been crushed, vaporized, distilled, and recombined into a dizzying array of novel intoxicants.

The experiences that chemists have cooked up include MDMA and LSD, which were so exciting and unusual that they spawned entire cultural movements. Scientists have also produced some terrible train wrecks. Diamorphine was originally conceived as a non-addictive form of morphine, but heroin, as it is more commonly known, is anything but. Attempts at synthetic opiates have spawned even worse, in the forms of fentanyl and desomorphine, also known as krokodil, the corrosive scourge of Eastern Europe.

But if we can use science to consign deadly diseases to history, trigger the immune system to fight cancer, and find ways to communicate with people in semi-vegetative states, surely we can create drugs that satisfy our thirst for an enhanced experience without dragging us into the pits of hangovers, dependence, addiction, or psychosis.

Of course, there is no such thing as *the* ideal drug. Everyone is different, and when it comes to neurochemistry there will never be a "one size fits all" solution. Some like uppers, others prefer downers, and still others are fond of a "sideways." However, there are a few broad principles we can apply. The designer drug of our dreams would not be addictive. It would not produce hangovers, comedowns, or withdrawal. It would not be "moreish"– for example, LSD rarely spawns cravings as soon as you partake, unlike alcohol and nicotine. It would not have a high "tolerance profile," meaning one won't rapidly require a stronger dose to feel the effects. And it wouldn't bring ravaging side effects, from weakened livers to temporary psychosis.

Three factors determine a drug's potential for abuse, says Adam Winstock, an addiction medicine specialist at University College London and founder of the Global Drug Survey, an annual assessment of the world's drug habits. Those factors are the speed of onset, the intensity, and the duration. "What you really want in a drug is the ability to adjust those three things," he says. The chemists of the future should keep those three factors in mind to create a drug that is "modifiable," he says.

With drugs that are flexible in their speed of onset, people could move into their state of intoxication quickly or slowly, depending on their mood and their plans. You also want to be able to "titrate" the intensity of the dose. Booze is under a lot of fire these days for its health impacts, but from a titration perspective it's great: You can have a lot to get hammered quickly, or consume it at a leisurely pace for a whole day. Ketamine in tiny doses feels like being very drunk, but in large amounts it leads to a full-blown psychedelic experience that is off the charts. LSD, on the other hand, is pretty much a binary experience: you're either in or out.

Drugs that last an excessively long time are also undesirable. "If you only have three or four hours to spare, you want to be able to recover quickly," Winstock says. That makes 2C-B or psilocybin more favorable than LSD, for example. Nitrous, though it's extremely "moreish" (hence the nickname "hippie crack") has a profoundly rapid recovery time, making it a fantastic anesthetic.

The technology used to administer drugs is also a key thing to consider–and we've seen huge changes in the past five years. "Vaping is the biggest change in the route of delivery since the development of the hypodermic needle," says Winstock. There's also now a legal intranasal device for snorting esketamine (a relative of regular old ketamine) for use as an antidepressant. "I can imagine there could be new forms of vaping and aerosols to allow the absorption of drugs in order to avoid harm to the lungs, akin to asthma inhalers," he says. "I could also imagine transdermal patches that deliver a drug in a nice, slow, constant dose throughout the day, like an MDMA patch."

And maybe most important: new and better antidotes. "People need something to bring you down now and sober you up immediately but is less brutal than naloxone," Winstock says, referring to a chemical delivered by paramedics to block the effects of opioids and save people from dying of overdose.

Drugs with cleaner delivery methods, effective prophylactics and antidotes, and optimal intensity, duration, and speed of onset would all be helpful. But what would an ideal drug *feel* like?

Fictitious drugs tell us a great deal about what the human heart desires. The "soma" of Aldous Huxley's Brave New World sounds an awful lot like an opioid (without the withdrawal) or a benzo like Valium: safe, warm, carefree. The "Drink Me" concoction of Lewis Carroll's *Alice In Wonderland*—with the capacity to bend spatial perception and your relation to your body—certainly resembles LSD (though that drug did not exist when Carroll wrote his tale). And then there's the "mélange," aka "the spice," in Frank Herbert's *Dune*. In tiny doses, it produces heightened awareness. In big ones, it creates an experience so full-blown it can allow interstellar travel. It is literally a trip. The big problem with that fictional drug: it's highly addictive, and withdrawal can be fatal.

So if we put it all together, combining properties that are desirable with experiential qualities we know people would want, what would be the most tantalizing possible new intoxicant?

For my money, I'd say put a powerful psychedelic like psilocybin or DMT into a device like an asthma inhaler, which is even safer than vaping. I'd want two settings: volume and duration, so I could choose how intense the high could be and for how long. Have just a bit and you feel sparkly; a huge amount and the world melts. And by setting the time meter, I could come back sober *exactly* when I want to. It's no fun waking up for work the next day and still not feeling with it.

Then again, Mike Jay, author of several books about drugs, including *Emperors of Dreams*, which describes Victorian-era crazes, suggests the next great drug doesn't even need to be created. He thinks we aren't fully exploiting what's already available naturally.

"We've prohibited a lot of great substances which have been traditionally consumed around the world and which have great potential, but which are sitting around unused in the West because nobody knows about them due to drug prohibition," he says. "A lot of the frenetic desire to design new drugs is because the good ones are banned."

Top of his list is kava, the milky, warm, evening drink consumed by people in the Pacific islands. It's legal in the U.S. and illegal in Europe, but either way we've never created a good market for it, he says. "Which is a shame," he says. "It gives you a nice, brief, euphoric buzz. It has an effect that is a bit like an herbal Valium: you sleep very well, but unlike Valium, there's no dependency. I'm a great fan of it. They have some kava products in America, but none of them are any good. You need to use the raw root grown in the tropics of the South Pacific."

As for stimulants, coca tea—the traditional daily tonic for people in the high-elevation climates of the Andes—is a great upper, he says. "As a stimulant, I think it's much better than caffeine: people don't use it to get high, but for working, walking, endurance. It's great for things like gardening, driving—activities that require a bit of focus, concentration, and energy," he says. "If you want a slow release that is long-acting, you don't need to invent a new stimulant. We've had these naturally occurring drugs for 10,000 years."

Lux Alptraum

The Perfect Orgasm

The Perfect Orgasm

Lux Alptraum, the former editor of Fleshbot, is the author of *Faking It: The Lies Women Tell About Sex—and the Truths They Reveal*. She writes a weekly column about sex and technology for OneZero.

For more than a decade, I've been writing about, reviewing, and helping to develop sex toys. Over and over again, people give me the same idea for the future of sex tech.

To put it simply, they imagine a sex toy that takes all of the work out of self pleasure, a device that—via some combination of robotics, biodata, and machine learning—monitors your body to assess your level of arousal, and adapts its behavior accordingly. It would guarantee the ultimate orgasm every time.

It's easy to understand why this idea is so alluring; why a crowdfunding campaign advertising itself as "the first artificially intelligent vibrator" attracted the attention of *The View*, why the press eats up white papers that claim to map out a path toward smarter sex toys, why I've wound up in so many design meetings where someone tells me about their great new plan for a vibrator that will figure out exactly what you like. Sexual pleasure is notoriously tricky. It can be difficult enough to assess what feels good, or how we want to be pleasured; to then put those desires into words and communicate them to a partner can feel formidable, if not outright impossible.

A device that can cut through all of that, relying on the secret language of the body to determine our sexual desires for us, promises to bring us to the heights of pleasure without ever asking us to lift a finger (both literally and figuratively). It's a device that promises to unlock our sexual potential without requiring us to unscramble the confusing and sometimes conflicting messages our body provides our brain about what we do and don't want during sex. Of course it sounds appealing—particularly to anyone looking to profit off other people's sexual pleasure.

But I don't think we'd actually be that enamored with this fantasy if it ever came true. Like so many of our erotic imaginings, this idea is likely the hottest when it remains a possibility rather than a reality.

Despite the hunch that our biodata can be decoded to tell a detailed story about our arousal patterns and desires, research suggests that the relationship between our physical signs of arousal and our brain's perception of pleasure isn't as straightforward as we might like to think. A penis may swell, or a vagina may lubricate, without our brains feeling the least bit aroused; even orgasm isn't guaranteed to be an experience that registers as purely pleasurable. If there's no direct connection between what our body is doing and how our brains feel, it's hard to imagine that a sex toy might be able to figure out what we *really* want purely based on our physical response.

And most importantly, as appealing as an effortless orgasm might sound, I'm doubtful that it would truly be exciting. Sexuality, and sexual pleasure, are about more than merely arriving at an explosive endpoint. They're a lifelong journey of self understanding and self exploration, and the struggle for knowledge is as important as the ultimate destination.

A sex toy that promises to effortlessly guide us to peaks of erotic enjoyment may seem like the epitome of erotic experience. But in reality, it'd be more like a cheap trick that cheats us out of some of the very best parts of sex.

The best sex toys integrate right into the sex we're already engaging in, enhancing our pleasure without making themselves the main attraction. When I envision the future of sex toys, I see products that are effortless to charge (or never need charging at all), easy to clean, ergonomic, and affordable. All we really need are simple products that do more by doing less.

Hannu Rajaniemi

Vanilla Memories

Vanilla Memories

Hannu Rajaniemi is the author of several science-fiction novels, including *The Quantum Thief*, *Summerland*, and the upcoming synbio-themed *Darkome*. He is cofounder and CEO of HelixNano, which is developing novel cancer treatments.

Part One

Two days after the CDC travel ban was lifted, Edie Ribas came home to Winters to see her parents.

The self-drive took her past endless fields of wheat and then the Winton Farm's neat rows of almond trees. She opened the window and breathed in the smell of dung and sun and dust. It could have been the day she left for college, 10 years ago. The only difference was the eerie silence. It sat heavy in her chest as the car came to a halt on the gravelly driveway of her parents' farm.

She had spent the journey from San Francisco eyeflicking through wiki pages in her iGlasses on how to deal with the Infected, telling herself it was going to be fine. The gene edits in the Altruists' virus affected everybody slightly differently. Mom and Dad had been a little quiet but more or less normal in their brief holocalls during the quarantine. Still, one thing had stood out of the chorus of contradictory Internet advice.

You couldn't really tell until you met the Infected in person.

Low fences and trees made the farm into a labyrinth that had been the perfect playground when Edie was growing up. Besides the house, there was a barn, two cottages, and of course the greenhouse. The glamping teepees were later additions for the Airbnb guests drawn to the place's quirky layout, the Central Valley sun, and her mother's zoo of mostly unfinished junk metal sculptures. The row of rusty robots by the main entrance were still missing arms and legs.

Edie rang the doorbell. No one answered, but a fierce yapping started behind the door. She smiled. Snow had been a puppy when she'd left, but the sound was achingly familiar.

She bent over and felt beneath a broken pot in the bed of salvia that lined the path to the house. The spare key was still there. Edie unlocked the door. The small, scrappy dog stormed out, did a little dance, and dropped a battered tennis ball at her feet.

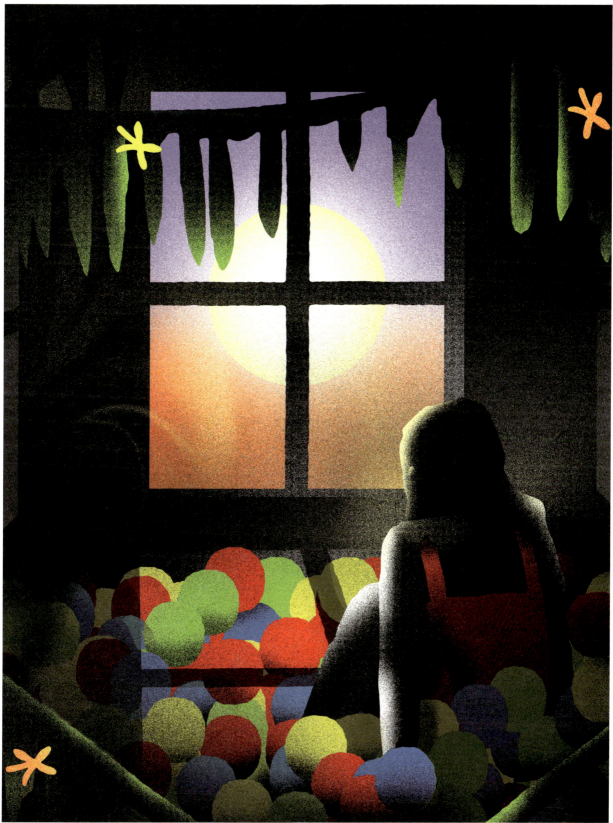

Illustration by Daniel Zender

She scratched his ears, picked up the ball, and went inside.

She made her way through the quiet house, the dog following at her heels. Supposedly the Infected stopped caring about trivialities like house cleaning, but everything was just like she remembered. In the kitchen, the dishes were piled neatly by the sink. A faint metallic clanging in the distance explained her parents' absence. Mom was working–and she could guess where Dad was. Edie followed the sound through the back door.

She found her mother behind the barn, making a metal tree.

June Ribas's diminutive frame was almost completely swallowed by an industrial exo-skeleton. She used one of the hydraulic frame's bright yellow claws to hold a giant silvery branch against an oversized anvil while hammering at it with rapid, precise blows. The branch clearly belonged to the larger piece that loomed behind Edie's mother. It was a mass of interwoven silver tendrils that reached for the sky, at least 20 feet high. Every gleaming surface was embossed with intricate designs: faces, animals, landscapes.

Edie stared at the tree, mouth agape. The tennis ball fell from her hand. She almost didn't notice that the clanging stopped. June opened the exoskeleton's latches, stepped out, and took off her goggles. Her brown eyes were ringed with red marks, but the sheen of sweat on her face gave her a healthy glow.

Edie took an involuntary step back. Mom was a hugger, especially when they hadn't seen each other for a while, and it always made Edie uncomfortable. But this time June just stood there, face impassive.

"Hi, Mom."

June said nothing, only cocked her head to one side. Snow danced at her feet, offering her the ball Edie had dropped. Then it was like something clicked in her head, and a smile appeared on her face.

"Edie," she said. "Would you like something to drink? I'm sure it was a long drive."

Edie's skin crawled. She recalled that people with a neurological condition called Capgras syndrome believed that people in their lives had been replaced by aliens or robots. Now she knew what it was like. This person looked and sounded like Mom, but did not feel like her.

Then she noticed the pale burn marks on June's tanned arms. "Mom, did you hurt yourself? What happened?"

Her mother frowned. "Oh, these. Spot welding for the tree. I guess I wasn't careful." She held up the smartwatch around her wrist. "But don't worry. The nice folks from the CDC gave me this. It sounds an alarm if I hurt myself and don't notice."

One of the genes the Altruist virus changed in your brain had a silly name, *FAAH-OUT*. The edited variant made you immune to pain and anxiety. The Altruist pitch was that it reduced human suffering on a global scale, and maybe it did. But it also drowned out something that defined June. All her life, she had had a mild panic disorder. Taking Edie to school had been a major operation. Their holiday luggage had overflowed with clothes, first aid kits, and snack bars.

Being careful was who Mom was.

Edie felt dizzy. She sat down on a rickety camping chair nearby. Suddenly, she regretted not letting Zur come along. Her partner of two years had never met her parents. It was not that Edie was ashamed of them; she simply wanted to keep her worlds separate. With Zur, she wanted to be the Edie she had become in the city.

Zur hadn't understood. They had begged to come, until Edie got angry, and the two of them had a fight about it. Now she ached for the athletic nonbinary's grounding presence.

"Mom, how are you feeling?" she asked quietly.

June smiled.

"You know, it's a bit like after a vipassana retreat. Everything is bright and calm. I used to worry so much about you, your work, those girlfriends you never brought home. When you didn't call for a while, I got a little frantic. But now I understand you're all grown up. I don't have to worry anymore."

June picked up Snow's ball and threw it. The small dog dashed after it. "Are you sure I can't get you anything?"

Edie's mouth was dry. At least now I know, she thought. One down. One to go. "Where– where's Dad?" she asked.

"In the greenhouse. Why don't you go and get him, and I'll fix us some lunch?"

Part Two

Edie hesitated outside the greenhouse. Dad was stubborn enough to continue his family trade of growing vanilla orchids, even with synbio vanilla on the market. It was manufactured using genetically engineered yeast that produced both vanillin and the hundreds of compounds that gave the natural bean its complex flavor—not that Edie could tell.

But what was this new synbio Dad going to be like? There was a pit in her stomach. She had to find out.

With a determined jerk, she opened the greenhouse door. Hot, humid air rushed out. She peeled off her spider silk hoodie, wrapped it around her waist, and closed the door behind her.

The vanilla planifolia orchid grew vertically, and so the greenhouse was full of fake trees. They were mostly drainpipes wrapped with chicken wire and filled with moss, although Dad had also repurposed some of Mom's unfinished sculptures; spindly limbed robots encrusted with verdant sphagnum, with long vines winding around them. The vines were bare. It was mid-February, and they only bloomed in March. The flowers lasted just a few hours, opening in the morning and shriveling by noon.

The smell of wet earth and moss took Edie back to childhood. This was where she came to find Dad when she wanted to tell him about a book she had read, or to show off a new bot she had coded up on her tablet. He always stopped whatever he was doing and listened quietly. Edie learned to wrap up her story by the time a pained look of incomprehension dawned on his tanned face. Then he told her something in turn, usually about the vanilla orchid: how it evolved before the continents divided, or how it was the most valuable product you could grow in a greenhouse in California since the heat waves ravaged Madagascar and destroyed the world's supply of the vanilla bean. Then it was her turn to be bored, and eventually Dad sighed, gave up, and went back to work. At first, she didn't mind just sitting there and watching him in silence. It made her feel safe. But over the years, it got more and more difficult to explain her ideas to him, Dad ran out of vanilla stories, and finally they both stopped trying. The silence became more sullen. It lay between them at the dinner table and during the long drives to school, until she left for college. They had barely spoken in years.

And now, back at the greenhouse, she felt like a hobbit in Mirkwood: lost somewhere she didn't belong.

Something moved amongst the trees ahead: her father, misting the vines and the fake trees. At 65, Tony Ribas was still lean, but hunched slightly. He was like a zocata vanilla bean in the shape of a man, the ones the growers discarded: dark and dry and curled up.

He stopped, held the misting nozzle up, and looked at Edie.

"Dad," she said, her voice hoarse. She made her way through the trellises towards him, avoiding the hanging vines. "I came ... I came to make sure you were all right. Mom is making lunch."

There it was again, that crawling Capgras feeling, only worse. Mom had at least gone through the motions. But Dad just stood there, looking at Edie like she was an aphid that had somehow gotten past his fungal biopesticides and was making mayhem in the greenhouse. It wasn't the kind of comfortable silence they had shared when she was a child. It was absence.

He turned his back to her and continued misting.

Something cracked inside her. She turned and ran, tears in her eyes. She bumped onto the trellises, tore a forearm in a jutting piece of chicken wire, kept running, brushed aside the spear-shaped green leaves. Then she was outside the greenhouse. She ran past the old chicken coop, Snow yapping at her heels. Her legs found an old shortcut to the highway and she kept going, arms pumping.

She didn't stop until she was at the side of the highway. She leaned on her knees, panting, fighting down the acidic pre-taste of vomit in her mouth.

Then, with shaking hands, she put on her iGlasses and called a car to go home.

Part Three

Home was the Caterpillar House in the Mission in San Francisco. It was a Painted Lady, an old colorful wooden house she shared with Jorge, Zur, and Innocenta. They had named it for its bright yellow coat of paint.

Edie was still shaky and tired from crying when she got in. Fortunately, she had the house to herself. She slipped off her shoes and dove into the grown-up-sized playpen ball pit they had installed in the airy corner room. The familiar smell of plastic and the massaging pressure of the balls against her back helped a little.

Back here, her parents felt distant. This world was hers. Here, she was the Edie who fed knowledge graphs to AIs, played ukulele in a band, was a soulmate to Zur. People lost their parents to illness and moved on; this was no different. She would survive this.

Her eyes felt hot. She wiped them and hastily put on her iGlasses. Work, she thought. I should do some work. I wasted the whole day.

She held tight onto the thought and checked Workbase. There was a long list of new gig offers. Grateful for the dopamine hit, she started eyeflicking through them, trying to ignore the hollow ache in her chest.

Work had picked up since she got the Bright upgrade. The eponymous startup offered an off-label gene therapy that was originally developed to slow down neurodegeneration in the elderly but gave young brains an even bigger boost. It cost a year's wages in untraceable crypto—the legality of the whole thing was dubious. Edie could not have afforded it, but Zur knew one of Bright's founders, and got her a discount. She had visited one of the company's hidden but well-appointed clinics. An impossibly attractive nurse in a Bright T-shirt had set her up with a robotic IV system that let her self-infuse the treatment—a loophole to get around the FDA.

It had been worth every satoshi. Edie had come back with her mind on fire. Graph architectures that she had struggled with for months suddenly seemed child's play. She got steady work with ad hoc centaur teams that mixed humans and AIs, acting as a translator between the two. Lately, she had started to lose her edge—pretty much every techie in the city was now a Bright customer—but she had enough repeat business to keep going for a while.

Ironically, the virus that she had pumped into her veins by pressing her thumb against a touchscreen in the Bright clinic was so similar to the virus the Altruists used to spread their gene edits across the world that she had been immune to the Infection. That was why the big cities had barely any Infected. The people who could afford to live there were also the kind of people who got Bright upgrades—which effectively doubled as vaccines. After the Infection, it was the homeless and farmers who had the most cutting-edge genetic enhancements in their brains. There was a certain amount of poetic justice in that.

But of course, no one had asked her parents if they wanted the Altruists' gifts. The thought made Edie angry, brought her back to the mad rush through the greenhouse, the empty look on her parents' faces. She closed her eyes and rocked softly. The plastic balls rattled around her.

Somebody slid into the ball pit next to her, and a soft hand touched her cheek. Suddenly the world was full of Zur's coconut shampoo smell, and strong arms held her tight.

"Hey," they said.

Edie opened her eyes. "Hey," she said. "Listen, I'm sorry about–"

"Don't worry about it, baby. How was it?"

Edie let out a shuddering sigh. Then she pressed her face against Zur's shoulder, and the tears flooded out.

"It's all right," they whispered. "You are home now."

Part Four

"It was like they were different people," Edie said. Like always after a good cry, she felt empty and light. Outside, a blood orange sun peeked through the evening mist that flowed over the city's hills. "I didn't even stay for lunch."

"That bad, huh?"

"It's not funny."

"Of course not. Sorry."

"It's fucked up," Edie said. "I hope they catch those bastards. They had no right to do what they did."

"Maybe not," Zur said, in a strangely flat voice. "I mean, it sounds awful about your parents. But it hasn't all been bad news about the Infection. The fighting in Indonesia stopped."

Edie stiffened. "Maybe they stopped fighting because they all turned into zombie robots."

"I don't think it works like that. Or what about this homeless kid in the Haight? She's doing really amazing mixed reality art. I've never seen anything like it."

Edie twisted out of Zur's arms, almost stumbled in the sea of balls and managed to wrench herself into a sitting position.

"You can't be serious. Are you on their side?" What was wrong with Zur? Sure, they liked to play the contrarian, but could they not see this wasn't the time?

"Girl, like the man said, I'm not on anyone's side, just because no one is really on my side." Zur sniffed. It was hard to be angry at them with the sunset on their face like that, glinting off their dark metal earrings and countless piercings. "The Altruists may be dicks, but they have some pretty good bioengineers."

"Tell that to my parents."

"And what exactly," Zur said very quietly, "was wrong with your parents?"

"I don't want to talk about it."

"High pain tolerance, low anxiety, increased creativity, not much time for social niceties?"

Edie said nothing.

"You said they were different people," Zur said. "Maybe. But people change. How much time have you spent with your parents lately? How much of it was the virus and how much was just life?"

"Jesus," Edie said. There was a weight on her chest. She scrambled out of the ball pit. "I really don't need this right now, Z. I really don't."

"I just think you should be fair to them, is all."

"Fair? What's fair about bioterrorists scrambling your fucking brain?"

"What's fair about life? This is exactly why I wanted to come with you, to help you understand what happened to them."

The anger made Edie feel like cold crystal, brittle and emotionless.

"And what is it exactly," she said in a trembling voice, "that makes you an authority on my parents?"

"Shit." Zur massaged their temples. "I'm sorry, okay? This is coming out all wrong. Listen, E, they are still your parents. I know it's easier to be angry and treat them like they are dead, but they are not. It might be harder to get through to them, but they are the same people underneath, trust me. You just need to find a way to talk to them."

"And how the fuck do you know that?"

Zur took a deep breath. "Because I got Infected. A few months before we met."

Edie stared at them blankly.

"Remember Jason?" Zur said. "Cofounder of Bright? We used to date. Before the company took off, he spent a lot of time just messing around with synbio. He's not an Altruist, but he's really into biological self-actualization. One day he downloaded the sequence for the beta version of the Altruist virus, from one of those censorship-proof darkchain sites, and made a batch of it. I volunteered to try it."

Zur sighed. "I know, not smart. But I was in a bad place, hurting, and looking for a big change. And it worked well enough. At first, though, it was like being wrapped in wool, detached from everything. I kind of just ignored people if they annoyed me. But I was still me, E.

"It took me a while to figure it out, but in fact, I was more like me. I was braver. Stronger. Maybe it wasn't just the gene edits, but realizing that I had the stones to try them in the first place. But afterwards, I changed a lot of things. Got rid of my birthname. Moved in here. And then I met you."

They held out a pleading hand towards Edie.

"You got through my shell, back then. I wanted to come with you to see your parents because … if I could help you see they were fine, it would be easier to tell you about me."

"Easier," Edie said coldly. "That's right. You've made everything much easier. Have a good night."

"Edie—"

Edie ignored Zur and marched out. She went to her room, locked the door and lay down on her bed. She stared at the ancient stains in the ceiling, trying to see patterns, like she sometimes did before falling asleep: flowers, animals, faces. But now they were just dark marks, and made no sense at all.

Part Five

After a while, Edie gave up on sleep. Her temples pounded with fatigue. She was thirsty, but did not want to risk a chance encounter with Zur in the kitchen.

She pressed a pillow against her face. This was unbearable. It would never work between them after this. The only option was to move out in the morning. To an Airbnb first, and then somewhere else, somewhere far away.

140

She got out of bed, put the lights on and started packing, hands shaking, full of nervous energy. These days, she usually slept in the bigger bedroom she shared with Zur, and the clothes she actually wore were all there. But at the back of a wardrobe in this room, there were two large plastic boxes full of old clothes and knickknacks.

One held a bunch of soft toys her mother had packed for her when she went to Stanford. She had never been able to bring herself to throw them away. She looked at the misshapen toy cow her mother had made herself, felt a lump in her throat, and quickly closed the box.

The other box was jam-packed with old college clothes, jeans that were too tight, tacky organic display T-shirts. That was what she had to work with. She folded a few of them on the bed.

At the bottom of the box was a small leather pouch, with a thong so you could hang it around your neck like a talisman. Edie's father had given it to her on the day she left for college.

She picked it up. Something rustled inside.

Dad had found the description in a book about ancient Aztec traditions. The mixture of herbs inside the talisman protected a traveler who was starting a journey. The most important ingredient was called tlilxochitl, a vine with pale yellow flowers and black seedpods. Vanilla. The pods inside this pouch were special. Dad had missed them during harvesting, and they had ripened and cured on the vine for three months. They were frosted in crystallized vanillin.

In spite of the distance between them, Dad had still wanted her to stay safe.

Edie opened the pouch's drawstrings, lifted it to her nose and took a deep breath. The vanilla should have been intoxicating. But as always, she could only smell leather and air.

When Edie was 6, after an afternoon in the greenhouse with Dad, she had gone to her mother and asked why she couldn't smell vanilla. Was there something wrong with her?

Mom sat her down at the kitchen table and explained, in simple words, drawing diagrams. Both June and Tony carried a mutation in a gene called HBB, and had mild anemia. When they had decided to have children, they had realized it was a terrible dice roll: their kids could inherit one of the mutations, both of them, or neither one of them. On average, one in four children would be fine, two in four would suffer from anemia. And the unlucky one in four would have beta thalassemia, a horrific condition that would kill them before the age of 20, with a monstrous spleen 15 times larger than normal and malformed jaw and teeth.

Edie's parents didn't want to roll the dice. They went to an IVF clinic in Mexico that used something called a base editor to fix genetic diseases in the germ line—it was a molecular machine that could change DNA one base pair at a time. And that was all Tony and June needed: a one-letter change, the doctor told them. June read some of the scientific literature and was reassured that the base editor was much safer and more precise than the media-hyped CRISPR of her youth.

It seemed like everything worked. The clinic checked the edited genome of the embryo they chose, and everything seemed fine—except for one off-target edit in a neighboring gene.

In an olfactory receptor that detected vanillin.

Edie closed the pouch. Her parents had not asked for her opinion on the dice roll. She could not blame them: Why would they not choose a healthy baby over one with anemia and vampire teeth? And yet, sometimes she had wondered if she could have endured a few transfusions if it meant she could taste the farm's first batch of ice cream every summer; understand the source of the passion in her father's voice when he told stories about vanilla.

She looked at her life lying in piles around her and was tired of being angry.

Zur was right. Edie had closed her parents out. She had told herself it was because they could not understand her new life, that it was natural that they drifted apart. But maybe the truth was something else. Not talking to them preserved the Mom and Dad she remembered, like dried vanilla pods in a jar. Maybe what had allowed her to grow and change was the knowledge that they would always love her, no matter who she became.

Surely she owed them as much.

They are the same people underneath, Zur had said. You just need to find a way to talk to them.

To do that, maybe she had to change again, just a little bit.

Edie hung the talisman around her neck. Then she unlocked her door, walked quietly through the house, and knocked on the master bedroom door, heart pounding.

Zur opened it. Their eyes were filled with a mixture of hurt and relief.

"I'm sorry," Edie said. She took Zur's hand. "I don't care if you are Infected or not. You are you. You are a part of me. And you were right about everything."

Zur sniffed. "Thank you," they said quietly.

Edie took a deep breath. "I know this is a lot to ask," she said, "but I need two big favors. Is there any way you could ask Jason and Bright to make a virus with one custom edit?"

Zur frowned. "He still owes me a few. I was practically Bright's poster child, back in the day. What's the other favor? Code up an all-powerful AGI that serves only you?"

Edie shook her head.

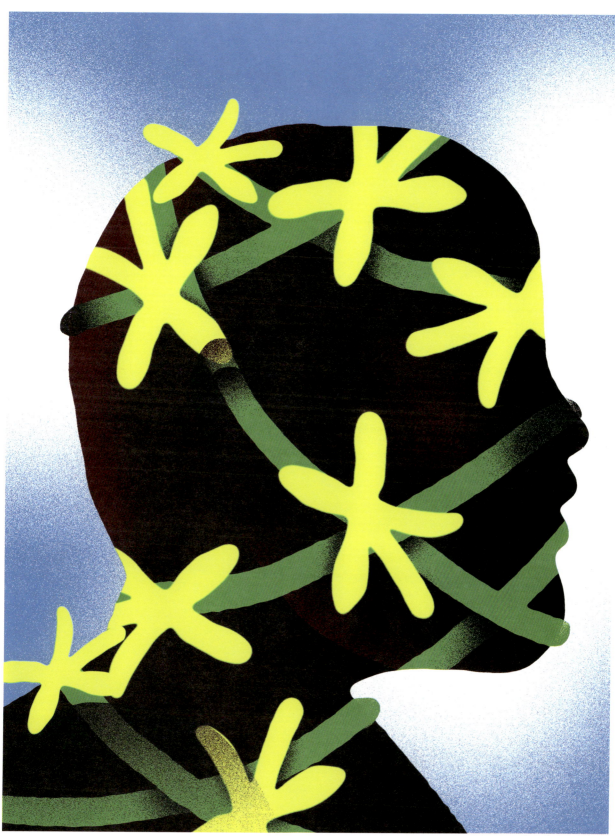

"I would like it very much," she said, "if you came with me to meet my parents."

Part Six

Three weeks later, Edie was in Winters again, with Snow barking furiously behind the front door. But this time she held Zur's large hand in her own.

"It looks like a nice place to grow up," Zur said. They looked a little nervous and had dressed up, in slacks, boots, and a half-cape.

Edie smiled weakly. She was on immunosuppressants, and the probiotic regimen to tolerize her body to the virus infusions had left her with a seemingly permanent stomach-ache. But today, that didn't matter. The March sun was warm on her back, and she felt light.

Her mother opened the door. Edie knew to expect the slow, alien look this time, and took a deep breath.

"Hi, Mom," she said. "This is Zur. I am in love with them."

"How do you do," Zur said, in a slightly choked voice.

Very slowly, a smile spread across June's face.

"I am very pleased to meet you," she said.

After the three of them had tea in the kitchen, Zur leaned over to Edie. "You go and see your dad," they said quietly. "I've got this."

The orchids in the greenhouse were in full bloom. The vines were ablaze with pale yellow, white, and green blossoms, larger and brighter than any Dad had ever coaxed out of his vines before. She breathed in the faintly spicy, cinnamon smell.

Her father was hand-pollinating the flowers, gently opening the side of the flower with a thin stick and pressing the anther sac and the stigma together with a thumb and a forefin-ger, an extreme look of concentration on his face.

"Dad."

He looked up, frowning, and for a long, wordless moment, Edie wanted to run again.

Then she held up the pouch around her neck, opened it and breathed in the smell of the vine-cured beans.

"I don't really know how to describe it," she said. "Maybe like honey and hay. Or butter-scotch. Flowers."

He looked at her, a question in his dark brown eyes.

"I got it fixed," Edie said. "Just one letter. But it makes all the difference." She smelled the pouch again. "It's warm, a bit like wood. And old books!"

"It's the lignin in the paper," her father said slowly. "It gets oxidized over time." He squinted at Edie. "You didn't have to do that."

"I know. I wanted to."

Dad looked down at the flower in his hands. He was quiet for a long time, and for a moment, Edie wondered if he had forgotten she was there. But then he spoke.

"I could never explain it to you before," he said, "but the best thing about vanilla are the memories." His eyes grew distant. "It was 29 years ago. Your mother and I were driving back from the clinic in Mexico and stopped at a gas station close to the border. It was a hot day, and the station sold ice cream, just one flavor, plain vanilla. We sat on the hood of the car and ate the cones, and knew that soon we would be home. And that you were on your way."

He finished pollinating the flower and picked up another one. "Anyway. Maybe you can make your own vanilla memories now."

"I will. Would you like to help me?" Edie asked. "There is someone in the kitchen I would like you to meet."

Joel Garreau

New Technologies Demand New Rituals

New Technologies Demand New Rituals

Joel Garreau, professor of culture, values, and emerging technologies at Arizona State University, is the author of *Radical Evolution: The Promise and Peril of Enhancing Our Minds, Our Bodies—and What It Means to Be Human*, from which this is adapted.

Once upon a time, driving through the drifting, eternal magic-lands of New Mexico, Jaron Lanier got to musing about meaning, ceremony, and ritual.

Even though Lanier pioneered virtual reality in the 1980s, he has always been more interested in finding new paths to connect humans than with the gear itself. Which is why he was reflecting on the time he was hammered by a man of the cloth.

Embryonic stem cells had come up at a conference at which Lanier was speaking. He recalls the cleric getting up and ripping into the panelists. "Even if it's just some little speck on a petri dish, if it's human, it deserves dignity and you guys are taking away our dignity—you're just a bunch of boys with technological toys. You have no knowledge of life. You are a disgrace," Lanier remembers him saying.

This denunciation started Lanier thinking. "I turned around," he recalled, "and I said, 'What kind of dignity do we care about? Do we care about dignity that is just granted? Or do we care about dignity that is earned?'

"I'm Jewish. If there is one thing in life that is not dignified, it's entering adolescence. So we have this thing called a bar mitzvah. The bar mitzvah is a ritual that is kind of a nuisance. It's kind of expensive. It requires a lot of people to participate. And you know what? It creates a little bit of dignity. Not always enough. But it does have a function. It creates some awareness, some community involvement and some responsibility and a little bit of pride, and there you get dignity.

"Dignity is something people have to create. So I said, 'You religious people. Instead of sitting on your duffs and watching us and then critiquing, you should be the ones figuring out where the dignity comes from for all this. I challenge you. I don't want to be living in a world in 20 years where there is a non-ritualistic way to do stem cell research. ... Actively create new culture.'" The most important thing is not to leave it to the scientists.

I like Lanier's notion. It resonates to my sense of human nature. If human values are going to shape our technological evolution and allow our species to prevail, we will need new rituals to mark our transcendence, to show that we're treating it seriously and taking responsibility.

The nice thing about ritual is that while churches can and should get involved—with their vestments and their sanctuaries—it can start from the bottom up. It can start with individuals and small groups, including those who describe themselves as spiritual, if not religious. They can take ownership of their future, and invite others to stand and witness. At these rituals we can deliberately seek patterns and tell stories—stories that might contribute to the master narrative of what is happening to us.

The beginning of humanity as we know it has been referred to by the German philosopher of history Karl Jaspers as the Axial Age, a period that spawned fundamentally new approaches to transcendence. Between 800 B.C. and 200 B.C., humans who couldn't possibly have been in contact with each other simultaneously grappled with deep and cosmic questions. All our major religious beliefs are rooted in this period. As Jaspers wrote in 1949:

> "In China lived Confucius and Lao Tse, all the trends in Chinese philosophy arose, it was the era of Mo Tse, Chuang Tse and countless others. In India it was the age of the Upanishads and of Buddha; as in China, all philosophical trends, including skepticism and materialism, sophistry and nihilism, were developed. In Iran Zarathustra put forward his challenging conception of the cosmic process as a struggle between good and evil; in Palestine prophets arose: Elijah, Isaiah, Jeremiah, Deutero-Isaiah; Greece produced Homer, the philosophers Parmenides, Heraclitus, Plato, the tragic poets, Thucydides, Archimedes. All the vast development of which these names are a mere intimation took place in these few centuries, independently and almost simultaneously in China, India, and the West. … The new element in this age is that man everywhere became aware of being as a whole, of himself and his limits. He experienced the horror of the world and his own helplessness. He raised radical questions, approached the abyss in his drive for liberation and redemption. And in consciously apprehending his limits he set himself the highest aims. He experienced the absolute in the depth of selfhood and in the clarity of transcendence."

Karen Armstrong, among the most eminent authors on the subject of God and religion, says of the Axial Age, "The search for spiritual breakthrough was no less intense and urgent than the pursuit of technological advance is in our own.

"That's quite endorsing, actually. Instead of seeing your own tradition as an idiosyncratic, lonely quest, it becomes part of what human beings do, part of a universal search for meaning and value. This is the kind of scenario that the human mind goes through in its search for ultimate meaning."

There is no human culture that does not incorporate some notion of religion. Even non-believers develop systems like Marxism that sport all the trappings of religion. This evidence causes Armstrong to believe that religion is an essential human need, as unlikely to be outgrown as our need for art. "Human beings cannot endure emptiness and desolation," she writes. "They will fill the vacuum by creating a new focus of meaning."

Are we due for a new Axial Age, an era of sense, intelligibility, clarity, continuity, and unity? The last time we had a transition on the scale of that from biological evolution to cultural evolution, profound restatements of how the world works arose all over the planet. Will something like that happen again as we move from cultural evolution to technological evolution?

In George Bernard Shaw's play *Man and Superman*, Don Juan argues with the devil about why humans insist on searching for meaning.

> **DON JUAN:** … *My brain is the organ by which nature strives to understand itself. …*

> **DEVIL:** *What is the use of knowing?*

> **DON JUAN:** … *To be able to choose the line of greatest advantage instead of yielding in the direction of least resistance. Does a ship sail to its destination no better than a log drifts nowhither? … And there you have our difference: To be in Hell is to drift: to be in Heaven is to steer.*

Perhaps it is with our rituals that we can start choosing to steer.

Right now the stories we tell do not match the facts. You can see it in the way we've handled our first primitive enhancements—our facelifts, our Botox injections, our Viagra prescriptions, even our knee replacements and pacemaker implants. We've been a little embarrassed about them, even while the number of new procedures soars every year. If we do not have a way to make them meaningful, are we doomed to be eternally sheepish about these lines we are crossing? Or should we start marking these rites of passage as an important part of the future of human nature?

Think about what happens when the first-grader whose hand you are holding is old enough to take her SATs. By then, there could be several means on the market to improve her scores by 200 points or more. They no longer seem remarkable. Those pharmaceuticals she takes? They simply help her express her natural abilities, you say. Like vitamins. They're no different from the memory pills the Boomers gobble up to banish their "senior moments." Her attachments and implants? So now she is always connected to Google.

Big deal. It's just simpler this way. Without her laptop, her enormous backpack bends her over that much less. She was hell bent and determined to have herself pierced anyway. Might as well have those damn things do something useful, like help her think faster. Hey, maybe these will help her get into Yale. Stranger things have happened. It worked for that babysitter she used to have, and he was thick as a brick. Now if they could just invent a new way to pay the tuition.

Can we picture rituals marking the great significance of a young person getting her first cognition piercing, awakening her mind directly to the Web of all meaning? What about a rite of maturity in which someone is formally recognized as finally knowing enough that is worth keeping that we mark his well-deserved first memory upgrade? Should we have a liturgy of life everlasting as a person receives her first cellular age-reversal work-up?

These rituals could have important content, important aspects of story. They could say: Never forget who you were, and always respect what you've become. You are a part of us, no matter how far you roam. They could include a formal admonition to use your new powers only for good. They could include the observation that we may be playing for the highest stakes. We cannot detect any other intelligence in the universe. Maybe that's because every other species in the cosmos has faced this transcendence test and flunked it horribly. This is serious. This may be the ultimate final exam.

Will these rituals do any good? Do baptisms, marriages and funerals—sanctifying birth, copulation, and death—do any good? My experience is yes. At the very least they are celebrations of transformation where people cross barriers of class, gender, region, race, and religion. They bring us together by officially marking and embracing critical moments. On these occasions, human connections that are rarely achieved elsewhere routinely occur.

If today we stand to transform ourselves more than at any brief period in our species' time on Earth, we are creating new critical moments. Perhaps we might start formally marking the occasions—marking them now. If we did, inviting those we know from all walks of life and all levels of ability to these ceremonies, it would knit together the different kinds of human natures to come.

It would be about creating the happiness of being part of something much larger than us. It would be about continuing to march up the ramp of human connectedness.

That, after all, might just possibly be the ultimate transcendence. It might be the point of this final exam.

Acknowledgements

The scientists, writers, and artists we worked with on this project—and many other people who have volunteered their ideas, insights, and time since NEO.LIFE's inception—have been spectacularly collaborative and enthusiastic about our mission. We are deeply grateful for their contributions to our still-evolving vision for the future of our species.

This book began with several gatherings to solicit input about how humans will be changed by the tools we're developing to engineer biology. Juan Enriquez and Nicholas Negroponte hosted dinners on the topic for us, and the Global Community Bio Summit at the MIT Media Lab gave us a chance to hold a pivotal unconference, featuring Hugo Caceido, Raymond McCauley, Lucas Potter, Juan Pablo Arocha, JJ Hastings, Beno Juarez, Abhik Chowdhury, and Elliot Roth, after which I decided to publish this book. The scenario-planning workshop organized with Hannu Rajaniemi and Zuzana Krejciova-Rajaniemi involved Seth Bannon, Rodney Brooks, Laura Deming, Kevin Kelly, Agnieszka Kurant, John Mattison, Ramez Naam, Megan Palmer, Lynn Rothschild, Peter Schwartz, and Christina Smolke.

Andrew Hessel is relentlessly optimistic about the possibilities of biotech and savvy about who and what to watch. Karen Ingram and Nicola Twilley had great and fruitful suggestions, and David Kong showed us how truly global this movement is. It's a joy to work with my dear and talented friend, graphic designer Jennifer Morla, and her colleague Reymundo Perez III, who gracefully shepherded text and image files onto these pages.

Laura Cochrane is the connective tissue at NEO.LIFE, bringing the people, images, words, and bits all together, and Nick Vokey has been a critical creative partner since the beginning. Lucie Parker at Letterform Archive offered a wealth of knowledge about publishing in the 21st century and crowdfunding book projects, while Amy Brand at the MIT Press has been helpful and encouraging.

What project isn't blessed when Sunny Bates helps out? Rodrigo Martinez, Iya Khalil, Robert Green, David Ewing Duncan, Agnieszka Czechowicz, Sally McNagny and the entire amazing MR tribe have been an ongoing source of knowledge, inspiration, and friendship.

Special thanks to Louis Rossetto for giving me the space to make this happen, and to him and our children, Orson Rossetto and Zoe Metcalfe, for their astute observations and never-ending support. We trust they and the rest of their generation will develop good technologies and make wise decisions about how to deploy them.

Brian expresses profound gratitude to Gretchen Heefner and Eleanor and Owen Bergstein. May they always be bold and curious explorers.

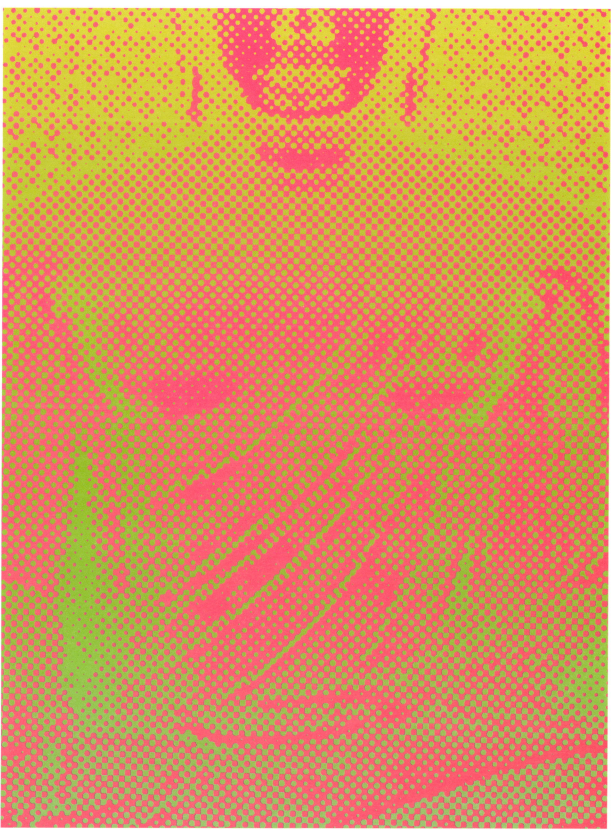

Illustration by Morla Design